DRY SKIN
AND
COMMON SENSE

by
Dale Alexander

DRY SKIN
and
COMMON SENSE

by
Dale Alexander

WITH ILLUSTRATIONS AND MENUS

WITKOWER PRESS, INC.
West Hartford, Connecticut

Copyright 1978 Dale Alexander
Library of Congress Catalog Number–78–50125
ISBN #911638–05–9

Illustrations and Calligraphy by Florence Valintine Omens

Printed in the United States by the Kingsport Press, Inc.,
Kingsport, Tenn.

To Trudi Semmel, my editor,
Whose inspiration, sincerity, and patience made this book possible. It was through her diligence, tenacity, and direction that my thoughts were brought forth with clarity.

Because of all her help and her devotion to matters of health . . . to Trudi . . . I dedicate this book.

Contents

OTHER BOOKS BY DALE ALEXANDER

Arthritis and Common Sense
Good Health and Common Sense
Healthy Hair and Common Sense
The Common Cold and Common Sense

Illustrations & Calligraphy
by
Florence Valentine-Omens

LIST OF ILLUSTRATIONS

FOREWORD

It is commendable to find a work that has such dedicated effort behind it. I can see that this book has been many years in the making. The research covers a long stretch of time, going back to the nineteenth century.

Dale Alexander has had to be steadfast against overwhelming odds combating trends that come and go in the medical field. One trend that is current and very controversial has to do with the subject of cholesterol. There is a growing misconception about cholesterol that Mr. Alexander and I stand up to. It is becoming critically dangerous because if the ill-advised concept is adhered to over a long period of time, it will have a devastating effect on mankind.

More emphasis must be placed on assimilation of what we eat. One necessary food group may be lost—even though it is in our diet—because its digestive partner has been omitted or removed by food processing or fractionation. This is particularly true of nutrients needed for skin and brain health.

Veterinarians have long known that the thickness and sheen of the coat tells the health. Dry brittle skin or dull dry hair indicates poor nutrient absorption. Dale Alexander tells how to obtain proper assimilation and directly nourish the skin.

Beauty comes from within. Skin beauty and health comes from wise eating habits—not magic potions from the cosmetic counter. The "COMMON SENSE" health expert, Dale Alexander, gives practical and reasoned guidelines that lead to healthy skin. This worthy book is written with great clarity and is must reading for all those interested in healthy, youthful skin.

Richard A. Passwater Ph.D.
Silver Spring, Md. 12/26/77

xiii

PREFACE

Over the years, during my lecture tours, I have been struck with the growing number of queries from my audiences seeking help for their skin problems. It is apparent they have been unable to find solutions.

The common complaint was that skin afflictions usually remained unsolved.

Gradually I realized there was a crying need for a self-help book on skin problems. A book that could show how and why certain skin conditions happened in the first place . . . and what can be done about them. The general approach from the outside has been wrong. It must be done from the inside.

My interest in skin developed accidentally. It was a by-product of my mother's recovery from arthritis. I wrote about this in my internationally acclaimed book, "ARTHRITIS and COMMON SENSE."

Her dry skin benefited simultaneously while her dry aching joints were being freed from pain. It was almost mind-boggling. Her new diet had a profound and beneficial effect on her dry hair, brittle nails and itchy ears. All this was telling me something. I had to write a book on skin . . . somehow all this tied together.

I was determined to thoroughly investigate its functions and dysfunctions. It has taken many years to acquire this knowledge. It became obvious to me that dry and other skin abnormalities are mostly distress messages trying to tell you something internal is wrong. The skin can be a reliable reflector of the chaos taking place within the body.

Medical research combined with scientific nutrition has given me the knowledge to put a meaningful skin book together. This book is not about techniques using creams, lotions, moisturizers that are short-term overnight cosmetic aids. All these are washed off, revealing still the same condition.

Because there has been a gradual but strong influence these past several years that we cut down—or—cut out fats and oils in our diet, people have been depriving themselves of oil soluble vitamins and essential fatty acids.

For that reason, I feel, there is now a greater acceleration toward dry skin, wrinkled skin and other skin afflictions.

It cannot be denied that an excess of saturated fats in the body can produce harmful effects. BUT . . . CAREFULLY SELECTED OILS AND FATS THAT ARE PROPERLY ASSIMILATED ARE NOT ONLY ESSENTIAL AND BENEFICIAL . . . THEY ARE ALSO NOT HARMFUL. In addition, these are crucially needed for the maintenance of linings throughout the body.

I have learned there is a LAW OF ASSIMILATION that makes plain common sense. This law is literally unexplored. Once you understand this and abide by it, the difficulty of handling the oil and fats in your diet will disappear.

"DRY SKIN and COMMON SENSE" is a book that will give you proper direction. May it bring you the skin health you have always dreamed of.

Part One

THE WAY YOUR SKIN WORKS

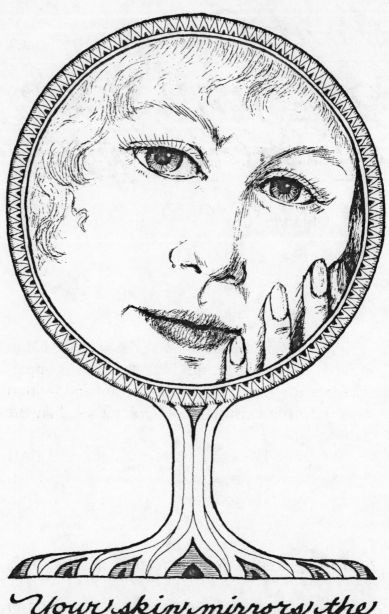

Your skin mirrors the
health of your body

At Last...
A definite way
to help your skin

The need for new answers to unsolved skin problems becomes greater every year. It is apparent to me that much that has been said and written deals with the existing problems rather than the causes.

You first need to examine the causes before you can achieve any lasting improvement. Then you can plan how to remove these troublemakers.

Learn Why Your Skin Has Become the Way It Is

There has been little research, if any, done on <u>why</u> people suffer from skin afflictions.

I have learned <u>how</u> dry skin develops. I have

learned how oily skin is produced. And I understand how skin can be both oily and dry. Then, too, I have the knowledge on why skin wrinkles.

I now know the basic causes of acne, eczema, psoriasis, and skin cancer.

I repeat, for you to know how to combat your skin problems, you first have to know why it happened.

For too many years, going back to Cleopatra's time, we have tried to correct skin difficulties by external methods.

The Great Skin Game

Some of us have paid hundreds of dollars for professional counseling by dermatologists, cosmetologists, beauty parlors—usually with ineffective results. Through the years, clever advertising by the cosmetic manufacturers has caused us to spend over a billion dollars every year—promising to deliver a "more youthful, less wrinkled, more attractive skin." This has proven to be an outright failure.

Therefore, I believe we have been misled. Attacking skin problems from the outside never gets to the root of them. We have been caught in what might be called "the great skin game."

What I will reveal to you will prove to be

revolutionary. The ease with which each skin problem can be resolved will be an eye-opener.

A Tailor-Made Guide

I have spent most of my lifetime researching medical problems in many parts of the world. Through consultations, lecturing, and questioning, I have investigated foods, eating habits, and nutrition.

Your desire is to achieve a better, healthier skin. This book will show you the logic of my findings. You have to know what your skin is made of, what it needs for nourishment, and how to keep it vibrant.

I will eliminate any guesswork. A step-by-step, easy-to-follow system will be outlined. This is a program that you personally will find easy to live with. It holds the key that will work for you. My dietary and nutritional approach is the correct way.

Here at last is a book on skin care that is a guide, tailor-made for individual skin problems.

The primary recognition in my lifelong career of studying nutrition and its relation to the human body dates back to my first book, *Arthritis and Common Sense,* which has been a constant source of help to millions of people. It is now in its

52nd printing and continues to sell, simply by word of mouth. Thousands of letters from readers tell me how my nutritional program helped their lives.

This book, my fifth, will provide valuable solutions for your skin. Fortified with the correct routine, results will appear, and most important, be lasting. Now let us proceed . . . to chapter two.

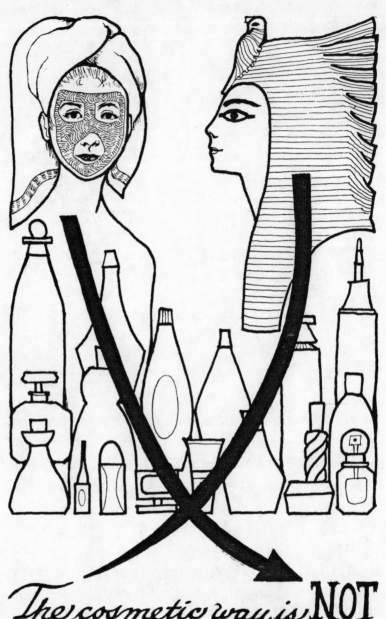

The cosmetic way is NOT the right way

2.

Cosmetic skin care

Employing cosmetic skin care in the search for true skin beauty is like chasing an elusive will-o'-the-wisp. The difficulty with cosmetic skin care lies in the disappointing result. As patrons of this cultish activity know, there are many contradictions that result in great confusion and frustration. This is not new—this practice has been around for a long while.

According to history, Cleopatra raised cosmetic skin care to an artform so as to stay young and alluring. She brought a sense of enchantment and glamour to skin care. To this day, an aura of luxury surrounds the seeking of the eternal "Fountain of Beauty."

Among her numerous skin beauty-seeking treatments, Cleopatra indulged in milk baths and anointing of the body with exotic oils. Now, at the risk of being beheaded, I think I would have been urged to tell her that her milk and oils might as well have been thrown in the Nile. Certainly oils and milk are good for the skin, but not in that

9

fashion. The skin cannot metabolize these nutrients the same way the stomach does.

The Cosmetic Scene

The Cosmetic Industry reaps over one billion dollars every year. It is thriving and growing bigger. Every day new varieties of "skin aids" are being introduced, mostly in this country and in fashion-oriented Europe.

There are cream and lotion cleansers; skin softeners (bedtime creams or lotions) ; stimulants (astringents and masks) ; protectors (moisturizers) ; and humectants (moistening agents; honey and glycerine are two) . It might be said there is virtually a cream or lotion for every pore on the face.

Compositions of So-called "Beauty Helpers"

Lanolin, a purified fat from the wool of sheep, is said to be similar to the natural fat secreted by the sebaceous glands of the human skin. It is widely used in most cosmetic creams and in many shampoos.

Turtle oils and creams are quite popular.

They are manufactured from oil squeezed out of the tails of turtles.

Estrogen creams are supposed to put back the hormones lacking in the skin. These creams are usually quite expensive.

There are a variety of oils which are laced with fragrances, and wildly extravagant claims are made for them and what they can do for the skin.

There are foundation lotions that are heavily laden with oils. Others are water soluble.

Masks: these can include mud, egg yolks, fish oils, herbs, and substances from foreign lands, such as pulverized rocks or earth.

The cosmetic field is an alchemist's heaven. There are no rules or regulations to check for purity or cleanliness. Occasionally, infections from a product occur, and a lawsuit is filed. But because most cosmetics are removed daily from the skin, these incidents are infrequent.

The lure of "quick beauty" is tempting. Women's "wishfulness" keeps the urge alive to try the new "secrets" continually brought forth on the cosmetic market.

As this book is being written, I am certain, there are new, exotic-sounding potions being concocted, hopefully to fulfill the dreams of some wistful soul who is craving a beauty miracle.

What Do the "Beauty Helpers" Achieve?

In chapter five, "The Remarkable Organ," it is made clear that the outer layer of skin is dead; that is, it is being disposed of every day. When you apply anything mild to the skin, it can be compared to a spray on your hair. The spray will not have any life-giving qualities to offer, since it is administered to the hair from the outside. So what you are putting on your skin as a cosmetic can be classified simply as "top-dressing." It is merely a temporary coating.

There are products which promise more than a "coating" effect. These are temporary wrinkle removers. Upon application of the specific product, the wrinkled skin will smoothen almost immediately, and remain that way a few hours . . . possibly for a day.

In my view, these products are of questionable merit if not actually harmful. The reaction that occurs so quickly can be the result of a mild irritant, causing a slight puffiness that fills in the wrinkles of the skin. The natural defenses in the skin will eventually overcome and weaken the effects of this irritant (if not too strong), permitting relapse of the skin to its former wrinkled condition. "Instantaneous" or "quick changes" should always be suspect.

The Cosmetology Salon Scene

One luxurious world exists for the affluent woman in the form of the cosmetology salon. Faces and bodies are heated, iced, cajoled, and pampered into heavenly submission.

But observations from some of the better-known establishments have revealed some directly opposing points of view.

Here are some of the conflicting pros and cons meted out to the patrons:

"Never clean your face with soap and water. Use only cleansing creams or lotions. Remove these cleansing agents with astringents."

"Always wash your face with soap and water. Use warm water at the beginning, then rinse and splash with cold water to close up the pores."

"Never use cold water on your face. Wash with soap and hot water, as hot as you can stand it. Finish up with at least 30 splashes of hot water on your face. This should be done so as not to seal in impurities in the skin, which is what happens when cold water is used. Also, cold water shuts off the breathing of your skin."

Manipulative facials are recommended by some and disapproved by others.

There is also disagreement over facial exercises. Some skin cosmetologists claim distorting the face with exercise will cause skin to stretch too much and create lines. Another point of view says the skin needs this kind of circulation stimulus.

Even laughing is frowned upon by some of the skin counselors. I know of women who never laugh. They allow themselves to smile, and only slightly, to avoid lines from forming on their faces.

The pH Acid Balance

The acid balance of skin is discussed avidly by some skin beauty specialists. These mentors lecture against the use of detergents and strong alkaline soaps.

Nitrazine paper is recommended to test soap and shampoos for alkalinity, so as not to strip the skin of its protective acid mantle.

The many different techniques employed and recommended by professional cosmetologists are usually gimmicks that are not constructive in overcoming skin problems.

There is one way, however, of effecting improvement in some skin complaints, although it is the last resort in cosmetic skin care. This is plastic surgery.

Cosmetic Plastic Surgery

Maxwell Maltz, M.D., has written a book called *Psycho-Cybernetics*. In it he states that cosmetic surgery is needed by many for improved self-image. This alone is enough to justify cosmetic plastic surgery. Unhappiness can be a true malady, and if the eliminating of a few lines and wrinkles or other unsightly skin problems relieves it, the money has been well spent.

Rhidadectomy (surgical fact-lifting), dermabrasion (harsh rubbing away of skin abberations), or skin peeling (acid applications) are some of the methods used in plastic surgery. Overhauling the skin by one of these drastic measures can prove to be very gratifying, but if the way of nourishing the skin is not improved, then undesirable and unattractive skin will gradually (and prematurely) reappear.

The Cosmetic Way Is Not the Right Way

The cosmetic body care approach is an endless and frustrating search. Healthy skin beauty cannot be slapped on as a clown puts on make-up. Beauty and health in the body shows on the body. The proper feeding of your skin will produce a lovely, healthy exterior that won't wash off every day. You will reap a twofold reward: inner health and outer beauty.

Many of the points brought forth in this chapter have alluded to, but not examined, the medical aspects of skin care. These are dealt with in more detail in the chapter on dermatology following.

3

History of Dermatology... Incomplete without nutrition

The medical specialty of dermatology has, so far, spent nearly 100 years in a period of trial and error. Answers to skin problems are not being found by these specialists—as they hop-scotch from drugs, to ointments, to salves, and skin creams.

So, let's take a realistic look at the science of dermatology. Here's why we are where we are today.

To understand the background of dermatology, I must describe four basic theories that fashioned the course of medicine. The four are:

1. Demoniacal Theory
2. Humoral Theory
3. Pathological Theory
4. Microbial Theory

The first theory—demoniacal—included the belief in demons, mythical gods, witch doctors, curses, and miracles.

The second theory—humoral—was based on the four humors. Blood, phlegm, black bile, and yellow bile.

The third theory—pathological—was, and still is, an important part of the diagnostic method. It is the study of diseased tissue.

The fourth theory—microbial—contends that diseases are caused by unfriendly microbes, commonly called bacteria. Louis Pasteur was the originator of this historic theory.

Through the Years, the Resistance to Change

There was much heartbreak and despair experienced by the many dedicated to making discoveries in the field of medical science. Interestingly, some of the greatest contributions to further the advancement of medical science were made by people who were not in the medical field at all.

Francis Bacon (1561–1626), English essayist, philosopher, and statesman, must be credited with introducing the experimental method. He felt man must have a truly open mind to progress.

He stated that "it is necessary to forsake the four 'idols' to which man has bowed down to, namely, authority, popular opinion, legal bias, and personal prejudice."

Galileo (1564–1642), an Italian astronomer, was the inventor of the primitive microscope and body thermometer.

About 100 years later, another man without any knowledge of medicine, van Leeuwenhoek (1632–1723), ground out by hand, an advanced microscope lens. His actual occupation was that of designing and making draperies to decorate homes.

He went on to be the first to explore microorganisms. When van Leeuwenhoek wrote a paper on the living organisms dancing all around in his microscope, the public was shocked. People were angry and indignant—accused him of making a lark of human life.

Next, we should mention Ignaz Semmelweiss (1818–1865), a Hungarian obstetrician. He became convinced that the unsanitary conditions in hospitals were the greatest cause of death for many patients. His use of aseptic and antiseptic measures in the wards under his charge resulted in a dramatic reduction in mortality rates.

Again, man's resistance to change prevailed. Semmelweiss' efforts to bring about the necessary changes in sanitary conditions were met with ridicule and scorn. This shocking experience finally led to his death. He went mad and died in an insane asylum.

A New Era Takes Shape

Until Louis Pasteur (1822–1895), the idea of infection by hostile forms of organisms had been entirely speculative. But with van Leeuwenhoek's microscope, man had now been given visual proof of the existence of the minute forms of life.

Louis Pasteur established the new science of bacteriology. It was this science that provided humanity with the means to understand and fight bacterial infection.

He was not a medical man, but his discoveries were of greater importance to medicine than any other of his time.

Now We Come to Dermatology

Dermatology—meaning study of the skin— did not become a specialized field until the latter part of the nineteenth century. This period was filled with confusion and disorder. The doctors worked independently of each other. There was no communication. There had been no common terminology established, no classification of skin diseases.

Dr. W. A. Pusey, in his History of Dermatology, said: "As medicine progressed, so did dermatology." He further stated: The living skin is the best field for the study of many of the important problems of medicine.

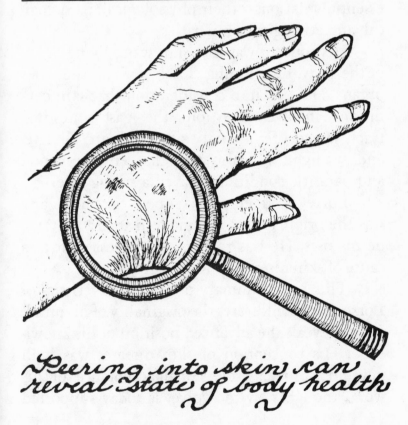

Peering into skin can reveal state of body health

I feel this was one of the most important books written on dermatology.

A Major Contribution By the French

Antoine Charles Lorrey (1726–1783) in Paris was a man ahead of his time. He undertook to analyze skin diseases by their characteristics. His efforts were to classify them on the basis of essential relations—their physiological, pathological, and etiological similarities.

His concept was that skin was a living organ of the body, functioning closely with all the other organs. He took into consideration that skin conditions involve digestion, the gastrointestinal tract, sexual life, mental state, food, air, climate, and sunlight. He also saw that environmental and parasitic conditions played a strong role.

Lorrey laid emphasis upon toxemias, and was the originator of the modern theory of toxic dermatoses. He was the first to suggest gout as a cause of skin disease.

This brief summary of the characteristics of Lorrey's work indicates the originality of his mind. It also reveals the advanced position of his knowledge. His conception of skin diseases was both new and broad. Professional acceptance of his work, though slow to evolve, is today supported more and more frequently as modern research progresses.

Next, Great Britain Advanced Dermatology

Robert Willan (1757–1812) was a pioneer in British dermatology. In 1785 he presented a plan for the classification of skin diseases before the Medical Society of London. It took him ten years to write his treatise on skin afflictions.

This work of Willan's was translated into most of the languages of Europe. The terms and descriptions of skin diseases used at that time are still used today.

He was one of the pioneers in emphasizing the relationship of industrial irritants as the cause of skin problems and other maladies.

He gave due importance to the roles of both internal and external causes in the production of skin diseases.

The work of Lorrey and Willan dovetailed to establish modern dermatology.

Germany—Its Impact on Dermatology

Meanwhile, Ferdinand Hebra (1816–1880) was at work in Germany. Students as well as post graduates interested in dermatology came to him from all over the world. They, as his disciples, spread his anatomicopathological approach to diseased skin.

He concentrated on pathologically-diseased skin, like tumors, infections, and psoriasis. He maintained that all symptoms of inflammation were produced in the normal skin by external irritants only. It was opposite to that of the French school of thought, which included internal factors.

Paul Gerson Unna (1850–1929), a student of Hebra's, made a giant contribution to the science of histopathology. (the study of the altered changes of diseased tissues). He gave us the method of reading the skin. He used stains to differentiate between healthy and diseased tissue.

Americans Then Took Action

Doctors from the United States traveled to Europe to learn from the experts there.

One of these outstanding Americans was Louis A. Duhring (1845–1913), a Philadelphian. He spent two years in Europe (1868–1869) doing research on dermatology. Upon his return, he became associated with the University of Pennsylvania—where a professorship in dermatology was established. He occupied that position for 35 years.

Duhring, in 1876, published an *Atlas of Diseases of the Skin*. His book, and his discovery of *dermatitis herpetiformis* (a type of skin infection), made him one of our nation's most respected dermatologists. He could be called the father of American dermatology.

A modern textbook available for today's practicing dermatologists is *The Structure and Function of Skin,* by Dr. William Montagna, professor of dermatology at Brown University. This book calls attention to the extensive structural changes which normally take place in the skin.

Dr. Montagna shows the skin as a parent organ with many suborgans. It includes the epidermis and the dermis, as well as the sebaceous glands, the sweat glands, and the piliary system (pertaining to the hair). Montagna has shown us the complete performance of the skin.

The Big Missing Link . . . Nutrition

I do not underestimate the value of these pioneers . . . or their process of classification and systematization. The combined work of these medical men and nonmedical men, the world over, was necessary to create the science of dermatology.

I believe that general medicine and dermatology have been treating what they see without delving into the internal cause. If research were done into the cause, then we would all benefit.

My objection is that we have stayed with classification, microbes, laboratories, and drugs. It is time to move beyond the diagnostic and temporary measures. It is through nutrition that we can secure lasting results.

I maintain it is a must to understand the total needs of the skin. These needs can only be met through proper nutrition.

Through sound nutrition counseling—with biochemical individuality in mind—a correct pattern of eating can be tailored to every individual. All I want to make you aware of is . . . that, without supplying the necessary nutrients, you are starving your skin. For the last 100 years or more, dermatologists have been treating starving skin with drugs.

This book will show you how to avoid skin starvation. You will learn how to keep your skin vital, supple, and healthfully radiant.

I have tried to review, in this chapter, the history of dermatology. Now, we have a chance to "put it all together."

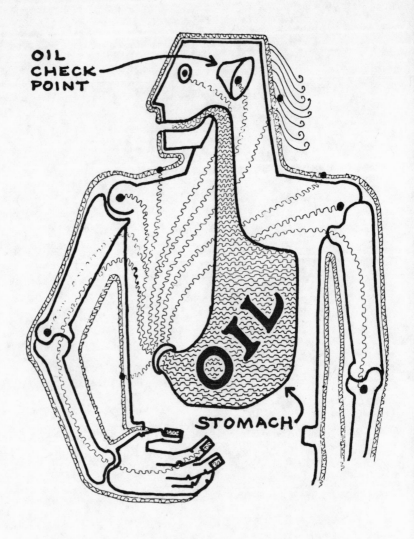

OIL
CHECK
POINT

OIL

STOMACH

The human machine can produce good skin given the right choice of dietary oil

4.

The human machine and your skin

Did you ever consider that your own body is a human machine? It has hundreds of working parts. Six of these parts—the skin, hair, eyes, ears, joints, and fingernails—have something in common. They all need **OIL.**

There has been an emphasis on cutting down of fats and oils in the diet. This has been particularly true in recent years. It has led to an oil crisis in the human body.

It is a well-known fact that proteins and carbohydrates, as well as oils, are capable of supplying fuel and energy. However, the carbohydrates and proteins cannot serve the body as sources of lubricants.

Oils can serve the body as fuels or lubricants. However, two conditions are necessary to permit dietary oils to lubricate. One is the presence of oil-soluble vitamins and essential fatty acids. The other is the route by which they enter the blood stream.

Therefore, you must select food carefully to make sure it contains oil-soluble vitamins and also the essential fatty acids.

Then the oils have to be assimilated in a manner to route the oil with its oiling factors to body linings, which are hungering for lubrication. It is through this lubrication that your skin is now able to produce that much desired element, moisture.

And if the oil also contains the high-quality, essential fatty acids, you now have a third benefit from the oiling process—the healing power within your body.

Look at Yourself As a Human Machine

NEEDS VITAMIN A OIL, AND ESSENTIAL FATTY ACIDS →	THE SKIN—Needs Vitamin A and essential fatty acids to give it moisture.
NEEDS ESSENTIAL FATTY ACIDS →	THE HAIR—Needs oil (from eggs, milk, cheese, etc.) to give it a sparkling lustre.

NEEDS VITAMIN → THE EYES—Need oil-soluble
   A OIL   Vitamin A—in pure oil
                         form, not in a capsule—to
                         add the proper viscosity to
                         the vitreous humor, so
                         that your eyes won't wear
                         out at too early an age.

NEEDS ESSENTIAL→THE EARS—Need to have
   FATTY ACIDS   high-grade dietary oils.
                         These oils will be used to
                         manufacture natural ear-
                         wax. The wax helps pre-
                         vent buzzing and ringing,
                         which usually precedes the
                         loss of hearing.

NEEDS VITAMIN → THE JOINTS—Need special
   D OIL   Vitamin D oil and fatty
                         acids from your daily diet.
                         They will create the right
                         viscosity in the joint cavity
                         fluid and help avoid ar-
                         thritis.

NEEDS VITAMIN → THE NAILS—Need oil-solu-
   D OIL   ble Vitamin D in the blood
                         stream to blend and regu-
                         late the proper assimila-
                         tion of calcium and phos-
                         phorus, and to strengthen
                         your fingernails.

The six parts of the human machine shown on the chart receive their sustaining oils and nutrition from the stomach. Since this book deals primarily with skin, where oils are needed, I am going to comment on how to select the proper dietary oils.

I will also discuss the equally important subject of proper assimilation. I will explain how food moves in and out of the stomach. How it then feeds the skin and the inner body—the linings, joints, arteries, veins, etc.

When the skin manifests abnormalities, there may be more serious health problems in the making.

The abnormalities can begin to show up very early in life—and worsen as we approach the middle years. Among these are such diseases as poor circulation (cold hands, cold feet, cold buttocks, cold nose) and blood sludge, arteriosclerosis (hardening of the arteries), and high blood pressure (narrowing of the blood vessels). One may have high blood levels of cholesterol and triglycerides. The eating of excessive sweets and unhealthy carbohydrates strongly affect the triglyceride level and could eventually lead to heart attacks.

Now, you can see how important it is that you pay strict attention to selecting choice and beneficial oils. After years of study, I have discovered a way that really works for you—and I offer this sound method here.

For the Human Machine the Four Best Dietary Oils Are:

1. COD LIVER OIL
2. WHOLE MILK
3. RAW EGGS
4. BUTTER (Unsalted)

Having shown you the most advantageous oils, let me take the reverse route and warn you about certain inferior oils.

Your diet is wrong if you consume margarine, hydrogenated peanut butter, bacon grease, meat fat, or fried oil. Avoid the fat from the chocolate bean, fat from inferior ice cream, roasted nuts and seeds, or an excess of any saturated fats or oils.

It is easy to recognize the symptoms as your

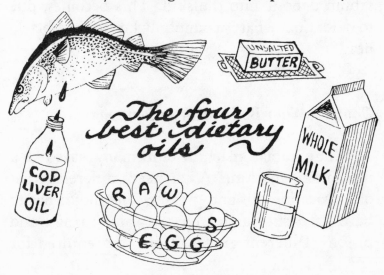

body tries to rid itself of saturated fats that have not been assimilated usefully. Examine your own skin surfaces. If you find excessive oils, they are being carried out through the sebaceous glands. They show on the nose, chin, forehead, scalp, hair, and with earwax that is too wet.

Because we have more sebaceous glands in some areas of our body than others, it is possible that certain parts of your skin can be oily and, simultaneously, other parts can be dry. Even with an oily scalp, you may have brittle fingernails and dry, arthritic joints.

Skin complications are also compounded by eating too many fried or roasted foods. Frying or roasting of oils literally plugs the oil ducts with their insolubility. If your diet has an overabundance of fried oils, there is usually an emission of sebum deposit into the skin. This becomes, due to oxidation, what is commonly known as a blackhead.

Compare Your Body to an Automobile

The human machine is in many ways like a mechanical machine. A car needs different types of lubricating oils and greases. The motor has to have its particular oil for the valves, rings, and pistons. Different grades of oils are required for the brakes, for the transmission, and highly finite spray oils are necessary to keep the squeaks out of the door hinges.

To meet requirements of good health in your human machine, your diet must contain a variety of oils and essential fatty acids. Well selected oils can keep your system working smoothly and youthfully. All parts of your body are designed to last 120 years, or six times the maturity of your bones. You should be able to live without the need of eyeglasses, hearing aids, and other crutches.

If you let your automobile wear out—owing to the lack of oils or the wrong selection of oils— then the car breaks down. Would you stop lubricating your car after the first thousand miles? I ask, why don't we consider the need for good lubricating oils for our lifetime? Is it any wonder we become dried up, wrinkled, and rusty when we get older?

Unfortunately, we have not gotten this kind of guidance. This has been sadly overlooked.

The Car Comparison Continues

Think again about your automobile—not only as it compares to the human machine, but how it also differs. Your car has three compartments (three pumps) to service it. One pump for water, another for oil, and a third pump for fuel. The human machine has only one compartment or pump—the stomach.

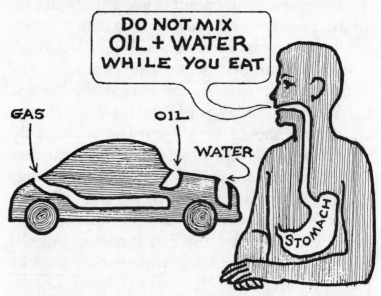

You do not combine water with the oil in your car. That principle, that oil and water do not mix, is the same for the human machine as for the mechanical machine.

Everything we consume (our water, oil, and food) must pass through our stomach to make our body function.

Suppose, by error, someone put water into the oil pump of your car. What happens in the crankcase? MOTOR SLUDGE. There will be circulation interference. The car won't go very far. Many things begin to go wrong.

You do not combine water with the oil in your car. That principle, that oil and water do not mix, is the same for the human machine as for the automotive machine.

When you want to know if your car needs oil, or an oil change, the service station man puts a dipstick into the oil crankcase unit. He can then tell you if the car lacks oil, or if the oil is dirty and needs changing. He can open the pet cock at the bottom of the crankcase. The oil is released, and then replaced with oil that is of the right viscosity and weight for your car. The car will roll on for many months.

How can you check to see if your own body has need for oil or for an oil change?

The human machine also has an oil checkpoint . . . and I will now tell you where to find it. It can be found in the external opening of the ear. Earwax registers the condition of your oil line.

Instead of a "dip-stick" you can use a Q-tip. By inserting a Q-tip (gently, not too far) into your ear, you can measure the oil content in your own human machine. Check both the left ear and the right ear. If your earwax is dark amber, cakey, scanty, or missing entirely, you had better take warning.

The evidence seen on your 'Q-tip' is urging you to change your oil, or add some new oils. You can only succeed by starting on a revised diet . . . one that includes the best dietary oils. It usually takes a minimum of six months to "change" the oil in the human machine before your earwax normalizes itself. If the wax is really dark, it could require up to one year for you to create a new supply.

Earwax can be a gauge to dry skin, the wrinkles of old age, the loss of hearing, arthritis, and many other problems.

Assimilation . . . The Overlooked Factor

No matter how many correct oil-bearing foods you have in your daily menus, they will not bring full value to your body without being properly assimilated.

To keep your body youthful and rejuvenated, the oil-soluble Vitamins A, D, E, and K are necessary, along with essential fatty acids. But even these will not do the job unless, during the process of digestion, they follow a certain route through your body.

I maintain that the secret to better health is to deliver dietary oils from the stomach throughout your system, but bypassing the liver. <u>Only oil</u> has the option of avoiding the liver just before entering the bloodstream.

Therefore, to gain lubricating potential it is necessary to direct the nutritive oils away from the liver. Once they make a circuit of the body, they come back to the liver. But, first the lubrication needs of the body have to be satisfied.

What governs these oils to take the proper route? The major cause is related to the liquids which you drink with your meals.

I suggest that with meals you drink milk or soup. Of course, we all need water. The time to have water is at least 10 minutes before meals, or approximately three hours after meals.

WHAT HAPPENS AT MEAL TIME

TABLE DESCRIBING ASSIMILATION PERCENTAGES OF OIL

A. If you don't drink liquids with meals.
50% equal distribution of oils divided into and around the liver.

B. Whole milk.
20% into the liver, 80% goes around it.

C. Non-fat milk.
80% into the liver, 20% around it.

D. With water, coffee, tea.
80% into the liver, 20% around it.

E. With iced water, coffee, tea, juices, or soft drnks, etc.
95% into the liver, 5% around it.

F. With Cod Liver Oil mixture.
None goes into the liver, 100% around it.

(Percentages are approximate)

Here are some advantages of the good as-similation of select oils and some disadvantages of the improper assimilation of oils:

GOOD ASSIMILATION OF SELECT OILS ADVANTAGES	POOR ASSIMILATION OF OILS DISADVANTAGES
	POOR CIRCULATION
NORMAL SKIN	EARLIER NEED FOR GLASSES
GOOD VISION	EARLIER NEED FOR HEARING
GOOD HEARING	AID
MORE AGILITY	HIGH BLOOD CHOLESTEROL
STRONGER FINGERNAILS	HARDENING OF ARTERIES
FIRMER BONES	HEART ATTACKS
STRONGER TEETH	STROKES
	HIGH BLOOD PRESSURE

Oil distribution, as just described, affects many areas of health. It applies to more than just your skin. It also affects all the linings through-out your body that need nutritive oils.

No digestion of fats or oils occurs in your stomach. The heat within the stomach changes all fats in your diet and converts them into oil. This heating process, in your stomach, requires one to four hours after a fatty meal. Remember your choice of liquids with meals will determine how fast the solid fats which you eat will be con-verted into oil.

The "heating" process which I have just men-tioned is another reason why I am so concerned about which liquids you drink with your meals. You must make certain which way the dietary oils will go. Will they travel into the systemic circula-tion around the liver, or into the portal circulation into the liver? This is discussed in chapter five.

You Are the Mechanic of Your Human Machine

I have given you a comparative analysis between a human machine and a man-made machine.

I have shown you some of the basic needs for a mechanical machine to operate well. I have also given you some of the basic requirements necessary for your human machine.

A mechanical machine can have a coat of paint to renew the appearance of its metal and it won't wash off.

It is nice that we don't have a cold armor for our skin. But we do have to know how to keep our skin soft, supple, and vibrant.

We human beings can control the health of our skin (as well as our bodies).

I have discussed some of the tested-and-tried information in this chapter. By reading the entire book you will know how to help your individual skin problems.

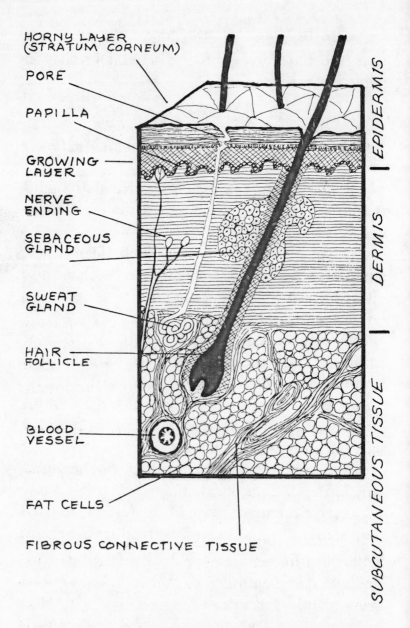

HORNY LAYER
(STRATUM CORNEUM)

PORE

PAPILLA

GROWING
LAYER

NERVE
ENDING

SEBACEOUS
GLAND

SWEAT
GLAND

HAIR
FOLLICLE

BLOOD
VESSEL

FAT CELLS

FIBROUS CONNECTIVE TISSUE

EPIDERMIS

DERMIS

SUBCUTANEOUS TISSUE

Cross section of the skin

5.

The remarkable organ... your skin

Skin is the largest organ in the human body. The skin of an adult weighs about six pounds. Spread out flat it could cover from about 16 to 20 square feet. It is the protective covering for the entire body.

This organ performs many necessary functions.

The skin helps the body regulate its temperature. Secretion of perspiration and waste material aid in this activity.

Beneath the surface of the skin, in an average square centimeter are some 100 sweat glands, hundreds of nerve endings, 10 hair follicles, 15 sebaceous glands, and more than 3 million cells. How big is a square centimeter? The size of your little fingernail.

The structure of the skin is composed of

three basic layers. From top to bottom: the epidermis, the middle dermis, and the subcutaneous tissue. The word *dermis* is taken from the Greek word for skin. The Greek word epi, meaning over, combined with dermis, formulates the word epidermis.

The Epidermis

The top layer of the skin, the epidermis, is made up of numerous cells that are horizontally lined, side by side, like cobblestones in a street. There are from 15 to 30 of these layers, one above the other. The cells of the skin grow from the bottom up. If we were to look in, with X-ray eyes, we would see an orderliness of nature.

There is a dividing line separating the epidermis from the dermis. This is a tier of perpendicular cells shaped like columns. There are round cells above and as they get closer to the surface of the skin, they gradually flatten out.

Evaporation takes place as these cells are pushed upward and outward by the new cells below them. Upon reaching the surface, they are shed as thin flakes. This is the dead skin a person often rubs off with a towel after taking a bath.

Skin is constantly renewing itself from birth to death. Billions of new cells are produced every day while billions of horny dead cells are shed by the body. Thus a human body gets a new outer skin every 27 days . . . the birth-to-death span.

The external skin has furrows and fingerprints that are uniquely stamped. These are influenced by genes, environment, and climate. These impressions are formed in the dermis and remain for the lifetime of the skin, unless burned or cut away.

The great master of all science, nature, equipped us with thicker skin on the palms of our hands and on the soles of our feet, obviously for more strenuous wear.

A network of pores is an important member in the structure of our skin. Through these pores a variety of functions are active when needed: for breathing, for secretions of perspiration, for waste matter. Body temperature is also assisted through them. Some of the pores are used exclusively by the sebaceous glands for oil secretions.

Then, too, external poisons can be ingested through these tiny apertures.

The color of the skin is determined largely by melanin, a dark pigment. The amount of melanin varies with each person but depends largely on heredity. Melanin is mainly a protective substance. It screens out dangerous ultraviolet from the sun rays. In all people except albinos, brown granules of melanin are contained in the deepest cells of the epidermis. This pigment is made in special cells lying in the upper level of the dermis.

The skin, when exposed excessively to the sun, is stimulated to produce more melanin. This promotes tanning and in certain inherited skin, spotty freckling will result. People prone to freckling are usually fair-skinned. They have less melanin and are unable to withstand much strong sunlight. They can easily get sunburned and are more susceptible to skin cancer.

I feel such heredity occurs when there has been a long-term lack of necessary nutrients. It is ofttimes repeated from generation to generation.

I know the way skin lives. The lack need not continue. The skin, so to speak, can be reborn and renew itself.

The Dermis

The dermis is made of a closely woven network of connective tissue. Its thickness ranges from one-sixteenth of an inch to one-eighth of an inch. It is the strong but elastic envelope that holds everything together. It keeps vessels, fat, etc., from bulging or falling out. The dermis contains a collection of intricate blood vessels, lymph systems, nerves, glands, and hair follicles.

The blood vessels perform herculean tasks, within this intricate network. If you or I exercise vigorously, the blood vessels dilate. We become flushed. Our skin is trying to push the heat outside to get rid of it.

On a cold day the reverse takes place. Our vessels contract, forcing blood to the interior of our bodies. We go pale. The rate of heat loss is slowed, thus allowing our bodies to withstand cold temperature longer. The purpose of this principle is to keep our bodies from freezing in extreme cold.

On the outer surface of the dermis are a great many tiny elevations almost two-hundredths of an inch high. These are called papillae. Their name was taken from the Latin word for pimple. The papillae fit into tiny grooves on the undersurface of the epidermis, and help connect the two layers. The papillae contain the nerves that are sensitive to touch.

There are two suborgans in the dermis. One is the sweat gland that pours out sweat. The other, the sebaceous gland, discharges oil. Each works independently. The sweat glands are isolated; the sebaceous glands are always connected to a hair follicle.

The Sweat Glands

The sweat glands are part of the human air-conditioning system. Their primary function is to regulate body heat. As the perspiration is dispersed, it aids in cooling the body. It is like letting steam out of a kettle.

There are about two million sweat glands distributed over the surface of the body. They are most abundant on the palms of the hands, the soles of the feet, in the armpits and on the forehead.

Each is a tightly-coiled little tube buried deep in the dermis, with a one-fifth-inch long duct rising to the surface. In this part of the human air-conditioning system, there are about six miles of ductwork.

Sweat glands function almost continually. They emit a salty fluid that can be likened to urine. The skin has been called the third kidney even though it is not as efficient in regulating body salt and water and getting rid of waste.

In ordinary sweating, about one pint of liquid evaporates each day. This process occurs invisibly and is aptly called "invisible perspiration." If the body produces sweat excessively, the amount given off may rise to two, three and in extreme cases, as much as ten quarts a day.

The work of these glands is governed by secretory nerves of the sympathetic nervous system. It is generally believed that a central sweat control exists in the brain. It is stimulated when there is increased temperature in blood going to the brain, or reflexively, when skin temperature is heightened. The rise in temperature of the blood is largely determined by external temperature and the amount of muscular activity. The sweat center is also influenced by nausea, asphyxiation, and emotional states, as seen in the "cold sweat" of fear.

The Sebaceous Glands

There are several hundred thousand sebaceous glands (also called oil glands) , and they are attached to hair follicles. It is their job to give off an oily substance that makes the hair smooth and glossy, and keep the skin from becoming too dry. The sebaceous secretion, sebum, contains fats, proteins, water, salts, and some residue of epithelial cells. This substance is designed to help preserve the physical integrity of the skin. Sebum also is greatly instrumental in preventing too great an imbibition (absorption) of liquids into the skin. You can comfortably bathe without fear of drowning your body.

There seems to be a general pattern in the way sebum usually appears on the body. The sebaceous glands are in greater preponderance in the scalp, the face, and in lesser and lesser degrees on down the body. Often the skin around the soles and heels of the feet is dry to the point of cracking.

The sebaceous glands are very active during adolescence. If the secretion cannot be properly discharged it lodges in the duct, as a "whitehead." The outer portion of this material may be blackened by oxidation and then it becomes a "blackhead." Their presence, contrary to what you may have thought, is not owing to a lack of cleanliness.

We bathe our skin with soap to dispose of an accumulated film of sebum and dirt. When we rub the skin for drying or for friction, we are ridding ourselves of dead cells as well as stimulating a fresh supply of lubrication. Through this process, with a sufficient supply of healthy type oil, we can constantly rejuvenate our skin . . . for the whole of our lifetime.

The sebaceous gland performs a very special role for the hair follicle. The follicle is surrounded on each side by two assistants. These are the sebaceous gland and a smooth muscle. When the hair is brushed, the pressure felt by the muscle forces the gland to emit sebum.

The Hair

Hair is an outgrowth of the dermis. The skin of the human body produces hair with about ten follicles per square centimeter. Added up, there are some 300,000 to 400,000 hairs.

Each hair follicle consists of a bulbous root, deep down in the dermis. There is also a shaft extending up and above the surface. Women and men manufacture about the same number, but the hair of women is often finer in texture.

Hair exhibits all of the characteristics of the epidermis; it grows steadily and dies after a certain time, but the root should live on and grow new hair.

Every hair grows as a blade of grass. The grass is ensconced in the earth and has to be cultivated with its proper food and water. Hair looks for its sustenance to a network of blood and lymph vessels. As hair is part of the skin structure, I know it can be kept growing with proper nutrients.

Subcutaneous—The Underskin

The subcutaneous layer means "beneath the skin." It is the fatty portion. As the cartilage cushions and thus protects the joint from friction, the subcutaneous tissue serves the skin.

It acts as a shock absorber to protect internal organs. Body heat is conserved by the insulation of fat within subcutaneous tissues.

Furthermore, it is responsible for well-rounded contours of the body. It goes without saying, women are more conscious of this than men.

The Remarkable Skin

Are you one who believes it is your inherent right to have healthy skin? Suppose you experience some skin abnormality such as psoriasis, acne, dry skin, oily-dry skin, or even wrinkling. Would you feel you are just one of the unlucky ones?

Our skin, being an organ like the heart, the liver, and the kidneys, often will not perform perfectly.

However, there is one important aspect we ought to examine. What makes an organ function improperly? Wherein lies the responsibility?

I will modify a famous phrase we heard from the late President John Kennedy. "Ask not what your skin can do for you, but what you can do for your skin."

Because we do not carry out our responsibilities, we are often left with high blood pressure, heart disease, cancer, or skin disorders. How do we handle these consequences?

For high blood pressure, we usually get a prescription of drugs or some guidance on diet. This usually includes a salt-free diet.

For the heart, there is emphasis toward the low-saturated fat diet and anticlotting drugs for blood thinning.

Cancer treatments can include chemotherapy, cobalt radiation, or other drastic measures.

Skin disorders are generally cared for by external methods. Creams, lotions, ointments, moisturizers, and even cosmetics are tried.

Specifically, we are concerned with skin in this book. Treating the skin from the outside, I repeat, is neither lastingly effective nor healing.

There is a prevailing tendency to relate defects in our health to heredity. It is true that we do have genetic strengths and weaknesses, and they can have much to do with how susceptible we are to infection.

In my experience, it is a fact that men, subject to male pattern baldness, have the option to overcome this heredity trait. They can reverse this by supplying the necessary germinating nutrients and hormone-yielding foods. This is outlined in my book *Healthy Hair and Common Sense.*

Your skin has been doing its best, waiting for you to turn on to good nutrition. It can still be renewed. It is sturdy and can last your lifetime without looking old. That's what makes it so remarkable.

The skin, because it performs so many functions for the body, is often looked upon as a complex organ. Yet it only needs the simplest of foods. The more adulterated or synthetic foods that are consumed, the greater the risk of skin aberrations.

What staggers the mind is the way this re-markable organ responds. You can make it healthy or unhealthy, just by your diet.

What your skin requires most is a common sense way of healthy nutrition.

Now that we have generally discoursed on the skin as a whole, it is time to take a look at some of the things that can happen to it.

Dry skin is one of the most common complaints I hear. The next chapter addresses itself solely to that subject.

Part Two
PROBLEMS
OF THE SKIN

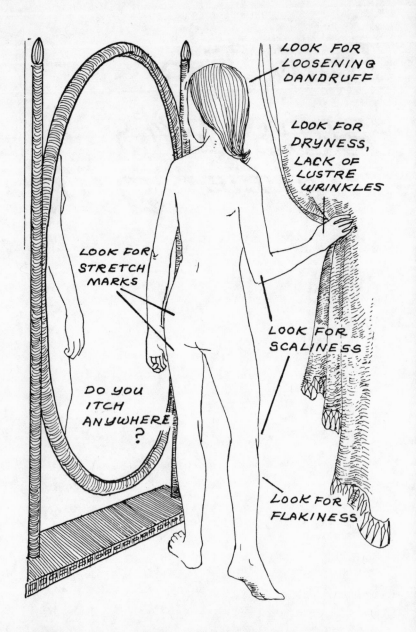

LOOK FOR
LOOSENING
DANDRUFF

LOOK FOR
DRYNESS,
LACK OF
LUSTRE
WRINKLES

LOOK FOR
STRETCH
MARKS

LOOK FOR
SCALINESS

DO YOU
ITCH
ANYWHERE
?

LOOK FOR
FLAKINESS

*Know yourself—
Check for dryness*

6.

The inside story...
My solution to
Dry Skin

The foremost problem for millions of people—both cosmetically and physically—is dry skin.

Parched, wrinkled skin is embarrassing and makes you appear much older than you are. In addition, skin dryness generally reflects other unfavorable changes going on within your body.

In this chapter, I want to make you aware that most skin problems develop because of internal causes. External causes play a relatively small role, even though most people feel it is the other way around.

Before I offer my solutions, let us investigate some dietary habits that can lead to dry skin.

How Are You Handling the Acids in Your Liquids? Is Your Skin Taking the Rap?

The skin is the first line of defense in protecting the blood from becoming abnormal. For this purpose, skin has a reservoir of buffer salts to counteract overacidity, coming from the diet.

Now for some transgressions that can create overacidity. . . .

There are different and specific acid levels in all fruits. When you chew a fruit, a process helpful to the digestive action occurs. The acid in the fruit is neutralized by the neutralizing salts in your saliva. Vinegar, also, when drunk, is devastating.

When you drink the fruit in juice form, the saliva does not get time to do its job. This results in an acid level that is too strong for your stomach's digestive tract, and later for the intestinal system.

Every time you drink fruit juices and they reach your stomach without first being neutralized, you are depleting the buffer salt reserves in your skin. You are stripping away your protection and making yourself vulnerable to dry skin.

Gradually, you may be subject to a whole variety of skin afflictions. To whom does this hap-

pen? It happens to people who are habitual con-
sumers of acid-bearing liquids.

Acids that are even stronger than fruit juices
are found in all soft drinks. They are never neutralized before reaching the stomach.

Taken daily, they can lead to dry skin much
more quickly than most other causes.

Another Skin Abuse—The Water, Coffee, Tea Habit . . . With Meals

The majority of adults drink water, coffee,
or tea with most of their meals. These liquids have
been discussed in many chapters of this book, and
how they disrupt the oils. As a result, the skin
becomes slowly parched over the course of many
years. Of these, tannic-acid tea is most harmful.

The Fat-Free Diet—It Takes Its Toll On Your Skin

It takes an average of six to twelve months
for a fat-free diet to produce dryness of the skin.
Scaliness often accompanies dryness when you are
dieting this way. I am referring to either a reducing or a cholesterol-free program. A brief crash

fat-free diet will probably not be hazardous to your health, but if this diet lasts too long, a depletion of essential fatty acids can lead to serious complications.

In conjunction with exposing the mistakes that dry out the skin, I am now going to discuss how to return the missing ingredient . . . lubrication.

How to Start the "Toning Up" Process

I feel the linings of your skin should have access, internally, to the finest oils for an assured lubrication and maintenance. Here are four high-quality oils that do the most for your skin. We will list them according to their lubricating potential. They are:

A. COD LIVER OIL
B. WHOLE MILK
C. EGGS (RAW PREFERRED)
D. BUTTER (UNSALTED PREFERRED)

Of the four listed, Cod Liver Oil, by far, is the best. It has a record for centuries of being a unique beneficial oil. You will read about this in chapter twelve, "My Romance With Cod Liver Oil."

Charted Proof—The True Value of Cod Liver Oil

Now I am going to exhibit below two comparative tables. I don't want you to get bogged down with them; they are very technical. I just want you to take note of the remarkable similarities of the fatty acid substances between the tables.

TABLE I FATTY ACID SUBSTANCES FOUND IN THE HUMAN BODY	*TABLE II* FATTY ACID SUBSTANCES FOUND IN COD LIVER OIL
Arachidonic	Arachidonic Acid
Oleic	Oleic Acid
Stearic	Stearic Acid
Myristic	Myristoleic Acid
Palmitic	Palmitic Acid
Arachidic	Palmitoleic Acid
Linoleic	Clupanodonic Acid
Linolenic	
Cerotic	
Alpha Eleostearic	Observe that Cod Liver Oil contains
Capric	arachidonic fatty acid, a remarkably
Lauric	essential substance. This is the high-
Brassidic	est rated source of Vitamin F . . .
Erucic	which is why it is the great healer.
Lignoceric	
Behenic	

After reading these tables you can see the outstanding value which Cod Liver Oil holds for the human body. <u>For lubrication and maintenance,</u> the linings of your skin should have access to this finest of oils.

* * * * *

Know Yourself—Then Try My Dietary Plan

Before I make any recommendations, it might be wise for each reader to do a brief personal examination.

First, look at the back of your hands. Look for dryness, lack of lustre, and wrinkles at the wrist. This proves an undeniable aging process.

Then check the back of your elbows and the surfaces of your knees. Look for scaliness at these sites, and especially for "Green Elbow."

Make a test for flakiness, by running your fingernails across your shin bones.

Check your thighs and buttocks for stretch marks.

Vigorously rub your scalp, and watch for any loosening dandruff.

Are there any areas on your body that itch, such as your ears?

If you have discovered any of the above symptoms of dryness, then you have all the evidence you need. It is time that you take action. You do need oil-soluble Vitamin A and essential fatty acids.

My best advice is that you begin, immediately, an internal lubrication process using Cod Liver Oil.

I have devised a way to make the oil most effective . . . and even pleasant to take. I call this the Cod Liver Oil Mini-Milkshake.

I have developed a process where Cod Liver Oil can be combined with whole milk. This mixture is more easily assimilated. It travels more readily from the stomach . . . and it is shuttled around the liver.

The Cod Liver Oil Mini-Milkshake is then piped into the blood vascular system of the body, where it proceeds to nourish the linings of the skin throughout the entire body

For maximum effectiveness, the Cod Liver Oil Mini-Milkshake should be consumed in the proper quantities on an empty stomach.

Your Blueprint for Correcting Dry Skin

Follow this set of instructions carefully.

1. To achieve the best results, take your Cod Liver Oil Mini-Milkshake one hour before breakfast. If more convenient, you may drink the mixture just before bedtime—at least four hours after your evening meal (or last food).

2. To mix and emulsify the Cod Liver Oil with whole milk is a simple procedure. Pour two ounces of whole milk into a screw-top jar. The jar should be large enough to hold four to five ounces of liquid.

3. Add one tablespoon of Cod Liver Oil,

preferably from the cold waters of the North Sea. Today, this oil has been deodorized—even glamorized—and comes in five flavors: mint, wild cherry, strawberry, orange, and peach.

4. Shake vigorously for about 15 seconds. The Cod Liver Oil Mini-Milkshake will then become foamy.

5. Drink the mixture immediately.

6. Do not take any food after this oil mixture for at least an hour.

7. If you are allergic to milk, or do not prefer it, you may use two ounces of fresh strained orange juice, to prepare the mixture.

8. It is important to use a four to five ounce screw-top jar. If you use a larger jar, more of the oil will be left clinging to the inside surface of the jar, and your body will receive a lesser amount.

9. Do not mix the Cod Liver Oil in lemon or grapefruit juice. These juices are too caustic. Whole milk, or fresh strained orange juice are the only kinds of liquid that are effective.

10. Avoid the use of concentrated frozen or canned orange juice. It should be fresh and put through a strainer.

11. Cod Liver Oil capsules are not to be substituted. The content of capsules is quickly captured by the liver, since gelatin promotes digestion, and the skin linings are denied proper lubrication.

12. After a while, you can start to taper down on the use of the Mini-Milkshake. After you see that the dryness of your hair or your scalp has been corrected, or when a normal supply of wax returns to your ears, then you can begin to ease up on your Cod Liver Oil intake.

13. Do not stop taking the Cod Liver Oil Mini-Milkshake suddenly. At first, consume the mixture every other morning, instead of daily. Continue to follow this plan for approximately six months. Then, the use of the oil can taper off to once a week.

Note: If you have a troublesome gall bladder, or have had it removed, use only a teaspoon of Cod Liver Oil in the mixture and take it on alternate days.

Other people who should deviate from the above rules are those suffering from ailments like high blood pressure, heart disease, and diabetes. These individuals may not assimilate oils very quickly. They should take the Cod Liver Oil every other night, or just twice a week.

Those with eczema, psoriasis, dermatitis, any type of ulcer, or skin irritation owing to nerve involvement, should use only whole milk to mix with their Cod Liver Oil. Anyone with the ailments mentioned above is often allergic to the citric acid and fruit sugar of the orange.

If you do not have any special affliction, such

as those mentioned in the above paragraphs, then
follow the numbered instructions.

THE RECORD	PERFORMANCE OF COD LIVER OIL
1850–1925 DR. L. J. dE JONGH'S WORK	RHEUMATISM, TUBERCULOSIS HEALING
1925–1950 DR. HARRY STEENBOCK'S WORK	RICKETS BONE DISORDERS
1950–1976 DALE ALEXANDER'S WORK	ARTHRITIS SKIN REPAIR

COD LIVER OIL . . . THE MATTER OF TASTE	
BEFORE 1948	NOW—BIG CHANGE
ONE FLAVOR . . . PLAIN	FLAVORS . . . PEACH, MINT, CHERRY, STRAWBERRY, ORANGE.
CRUDE . . . UNREFINED	REFINED . . . MAJOR ODORS REMOVED
TAKEN STRAIGHT: RESULTED IN BAD TASTE	TAKEN DALE ALEXANDER METHOD: MUCH IMPROVED— NO BAD TASTE

Worried About Your Waistline? No Danger!

After reading the above rules, and the story
of the Cod Liver Oil Mini-Milkshake, some people
will worry about gaining weight. You may fear that
this formula will add to your waistline. Not so.
One tablespoon of Cod Liver Oil contains only
100 calories . . . the equivalent of just one piece
of candy. And when the oil is taken on an empty
stomach, the majority of the Cod Liver Oil is used
for lubrication—not to produce energy or fat.

Instructions for
THE COD LIVER OIL SHAKE
with milk or orange juice

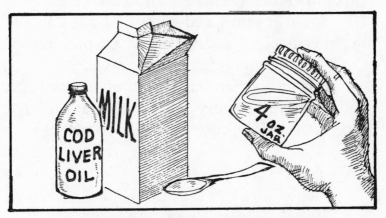

OPTION PLAN

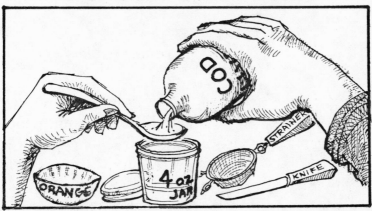

MIX TOGETHER, IN A SMALL SCREW-TOP JAR
1 TBSP. COD LIVER OIL WITH 2 OZ. MILK

OR OPTIONAL PLAN

1 TBSP. COD LIVER OIL WITH
2 OZ. FRESHLY SQUEEZED, STRAINED ORANGE JUICE.
(SHAKE VIGOROUSLY FOR 10–15 SECONDS)
DRINK EITHER, ONE HOUR BEFORE BREAKFAST, OR
FOUR HOURS AFTER DINNER, OR WHEN RETIRING.

Dry Skin . . . The Easiest to Overcome

You now know what to do if you want to be rid of dry skin. It is the easiest to overcome.

You will gain speedier results by also following the menus for dry skin in chapter fifteen. Draw on every helpful source possible.

It is much more difficult to understand how one can have both dry and oily skin at the same time. This will be covered in the next chapter.

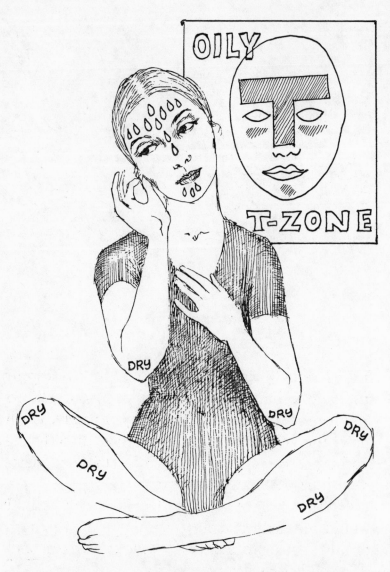

Change your 'combination'
skin (oily-dry) with proper
nutrients

7.

What if you have both dry and oily skin?

Skin that is both dry and oily at the same time, has for long been a puzzling problem. While your face and hair may be quite greasy, your elbows and legs could be so dry that they are scaly. Until now, the combination of these two directly opposite problems has not been understood, therefore, it has remained unsolved.

Since I have already discussed dry skin, I would now like to devote considerable attention to oily skin or to cases of people who have both skin conditions simultaneously.

As I do elsewhere in this book, again, I recommend self-examination. This time you should check your "T-Zone." What's that? Every person reflects, in their own face, what has been described as a 'T-Zone." It's an imaginary line, which runs

71

across your forehead and down your nose—where sebaceous glands are more numerous.

When too much oiliness is seen on your "T-Zone," or you have a "combination skin" (as it is sometimes called), it is a result of incorrect eating habits.

Be Aware of These Problems: Points Related to Excessive Oilness

POINT A—ADULTERATION OF OILS

The adulteration of edible oils has been accelerating rapidly during the past 25 years. In the days of our parents and grandparents, we consumed natural butter, natural peanut butter, and homemade ice cream. Superior natural vegetable oils were used. In those days, the body did not have to cope with denatured oils. Therefore, the utilization of the oils was carried out quite well.

The skin took, selectively, what it needed for lubrication. The inner body used the rest. If there was any surplus, it was stored in the waistline.

I have listed some of the foods below that create a hazardous production of grease:

Hydrogenated Peanut Butter
Commercial Ice Cream

Fried Shrimp
Fried Chicken
The Solid Fat in Meat
Pizza
Tacos, Corn Chips, etc.

The inferior fat content in these foods often surface the skin. If you do not control the production of grease, medically known as sebum, your T-Zone will be covered, and perhaps your scalp and hair as well.

POINT B—CONFIGURATION—OIL MOLECULES HAVE SHAPES

Every molecule of fatty acid has its own molecular structure. However, the structural shape of oil is altered by frying, heating, roasting, and hydrogenating.

The adulteration then makes these oils unsuitable for good metabolization by the body tissues. The result is usually that the sebaceous glands become plugged up rather than lubricated.

This condition is evidenced as blackheads (one of the by-products of improperly metabolized inferior oils). The blackhead apparently is the final development of carbon clinkers from the improper burning of the altered fatty acid molecules.

POINT C—SATIATION . . . THE SKIN OVER-LOADED

The two preceding factors, adulteration and configuration, are triggered by a third factor. The third factor is the age <u>when</u> you started these diet aberrations.

If you started these faulty habits during puberty years, you interfered with your normal hormonal balance. This invited a greasy skin much earlier in life than usual. The skin, when satiated this way, often leads to other skin afflictions.

Here are some more vital facts you should know. Edible oils in different forms are either <u>soluble</u> (unsaturated) or <u>insoluble</u> (saturated). If your skin is too oily, do you know which oils you should avoid? I have compiled a partial list, below, that warns you against some insoluble oils. The fats and oils from these foods will slowly find their way to your T-Zone.

"T-ZONE" TROUBLE-MAKERS

Margarine
French Fries
Potato Chips
Roasted Nuts and Peanuts
Bacon
Cold Cuts (Salami, Bologna, Frankfurters)
Hydrogenated Peanut Butter

Commercial Ice Cream
Fried Shrimp
Fried Chicken
Pizza
Tacos, Corn Chips, etc.

The fat content in the foods listed above has been rendered insoluble. You must eliminate these types of oils from your diet. Otherwise you will be producing a greasy sebum instead of a quality skin lubricant.

Sebum is the medical term for oils produced by the sebaceous glands. This is a heavyweight type of oil, produced from interior oils. When the diet is correct, the sebaceous glands produce a lightweight lubricant.

Sebum can cover not only your T-Zone, but your scalp and hair as well.

The Principle of "Double Bond Exchange"

The dry-oily skin combination shows an imbalance. There is starvation . . . and . . . flooding of oils simultaneously. Some parts of your skin are parched for oil. Other parts are flooded with oil.

There is one solution, if you are willing to take immediate action. I will now explain the technique in detail.

By consuming foods charged with high-quality dietary oils, you are triggering off an action which is called *Double Bond Exchange.* This is a term used in physiological chemistry. It merely means that you are exchanging high-quality, fatty-acid molecules for low-quality molecular oils already in your body.

Figuratively speaking, all unsaturated oil molecules have arms and legs. These arms and legs are made up of carbon, hydrogen, and oxygen molecules. The highest quality edible oils are of the unsaturated variety. Their arms and legs are very flexible and can interchange among themselves.

But . . . saturated oils and fats have arms and legs that have been stiffened by hydrogenation. The best nutritive oils, the unsaturated ones, can lose their value to your skin if you heat them excessively. This causes a structural disfigurement of the oil molecules. Their arms and legs have become maimed in this condition.

To carry out the *Double Bond Exchange* . . . you must first drive out the saturated oils that have "clogged" and "greased" your skin. You will start this by adhering carefully to the instructions for Dry Skin in chapter six.

The "greasiness" will be accented temporarily. However, it will gradually develop into a moisturized lustre.

For a person who has both oily and dry skin simultaneously, you must remember that this condition takes longer to overcome—twice as long as correcting dry skin alone. You are facing a long term plan, from six months to a year. That's what it will require to readjust the imbalance in your skin.

You should augment the Cod Liver Oil program with the Dry-Oily Skin Menus and food suggested in chapter fifteen. The menus work hand-in-hand with the Cod Liver Oil rejuvenation method.

This oil reconversion is the **DOUBLE BOND EXCHANGE** in action.

Isn't it nice to know that you can make a change in your skin simply through the means of carefully selected oils and nutrients? Your body, as your car, runs better on the right oil. However, there has to be a steady, persevering effort on your part to achieve results.

The next most worrisome "affliction" is wrinkled skin. Both men and women are often more concerned about their appearance than their physical well-being. For this reason, I shall devote the following chapter to the subject of preventing the spread of wrinkled skin and how to avoid it from happening to you too soon.

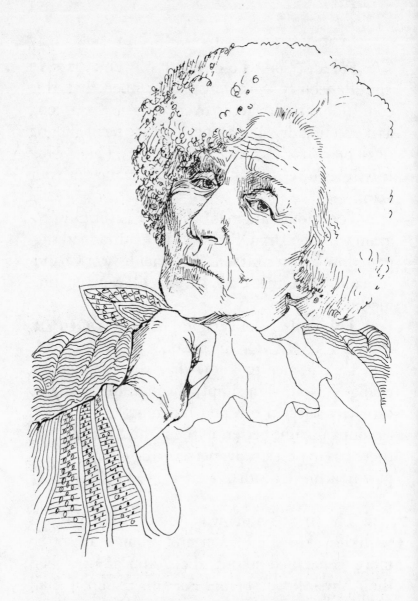

Dry skin is a forerunner
of wrinkled skin

8.

You can prevent wrinkled skin

The quest for a moisturizer, a night cream, a day cream, a lotion to prevent wrinkles . . . goes on and on.

Classes for facial exercises and books about facial exercises are being offered.

All this to prevent the aging look of wrinkles.

There is no end. Why? It is quite obvious that the majority of seekers have not found true satisfaction.

The people who have been on my program have found the real solution.

It is actually quite simple. First, you have to know WHY and WHAT CAUSES wrinkles. Then you have to know WHAT TO DO after you remove the causes.

True, it is somewhat more complicated than opening a jar and rubbing something on your skin. But instead of continually gambling on the

79

magic of a moisturizer, or a cream, you will be working on a sure thing.

If you intensely dislike having etched, creased skin, just read the next pages carefully.

Youthful skin—a younger appearance—is possible. Wrinkling of skin can be stopped.

First, you must understand a few facts about the composition of your skin.

As I said in chapter four, the structure of your skin is divided into two basic layers. One is the outer layer—dead skin. The second is the inner layer—living skin. To try to feed the outer-skin layer, cosmetically, is a fruitless effort. Why? Because all the moisturizers in the world cannot feed dead cells. It is senseless to try. This basic outer-skin layer, known as the epidermis, has no contact with the blood stream.

The older you become, so they say, the slower the turnover of dead cells. There is a war going on, in your skin, to remove dead cells effectively. When skin metabolism slows down, there is a lingering of dead cells. This can result in an aging, mask-like skin. If you do not take action, your skin is going to become starved, dry, and then wrinkled.

In younger people the skin has some advantages. Their cells have activity and are still vital. Feed the living skin (the deeper layer of derma, the inner skin) and you can keep cells from dying. You can increase the amount of moisture in your skin through nutrition.

Don't look at the calendar (your birth date) and blame it if your skin is aging. Look at your dinner table. Are you feeding the living inner skin with proper foods? That's the answer, instead of using cosmetic products to disguise dead, lingering skin.

If you don't consume high-grade oils continually, there will be a loss of elastin. If this persists long enough, the skin will wrinkle.

I repeat, it is not a person's age that decides wrinkling. It is the lack of high-grade oil being delivered to the oil glands in the inner skin. The skin can renew itself. But it needs wise decisions by you at the kitchen table. Correct diet must continue on a daily basis for most of your life. The effect is cumulative.

Remember that Word "Elastin"

Two paragraphs ago I mentioned this substance, and I would now like to elaborate on its importance.

The skin is supported by a connective tissue which is made chiefly of elastin. This is a scleroprotein present in the fibers of connective tissue. Supporting the framework of elastin, forming a glue-like web, is a material known as elastamucin. This is a polysaccharide-component of elastic tissue.

It is this elastamucin that is vulnerable to mistakes in the diet. My studies indicate that the drinking of tea, fruit juices, carbonated drinks of any kind, has an accelerating effect in destroying elastamucin.

People who drink liquids like water and coffee with their meals also destroy their elastin, but the rate of destruction is much slower.

Tea with its tannic acid, fruit juices, and soft drinks are far more caustic.

These liquids are indirectly instrumental in the wearing away process of the elastin in the skin.

How Moisture Prevents Wrinkles

Inside your own body you can manufacture the vitally important moisture to forestall wrinkling. I emphasize that your skin is like a chemistry laboratory and can keep itself from drying out. But, first, perhaps I should explain what kind of moisture you are seeking . . . and how the composition of this moisture takes place.

As I have said before, the oils gained from your food have to be of the best type to prevent skin problems. Chemically speaking, fatty acids are composed of elements like carbon, oxygen, and hydrogen. They come in different molecular shapes, depending on the source of the oil.

If the fatty acid globules (which have now become chylomicrons) are delivered intact to the skin, your tissue can metabolize them . . . and break them down into the specific lipids which the skin needs. Then, there is a release of oxygen and hydrogen. This is vitally important.

Releasing oxygen and hydrogen in this manner is what happens to the original oil molecule. The oxygen and hydrogen then recombine to form water. As you know, water is two parts hydrogen and one part oxygen. The natural oils of the skin then emulsify and help to "bind" the water.

It is this retention or binding of "re-formed" water which decides whether your skin will wrinkle or not.

By this method your body has created a new "dewey" product. Call it "re-constituted water." It is this new ingredient that makes your skin more supple and pliant.

However, if the skin receives oils which have gone through the liver, it cannot metabolize properly. The inner layer, the dermis, is unable to "bind" the water. Thus your skin gradually becomes dehydrated, scaley, and fissured.

Most researchers, and the general public, believe the problem is an insufficient supply of lipid substances to the skin surfaces. That could be true for those who eat an oil-free diet.

Summed up, I am convinced that it is a lack of water in the skin, rather than a deficiency of oil, which causes dryness and wrinkling. But keep this important fact in mind. The moisturization occurs as a natural phenomenon after the skin has metabolized the proper lubrication.

I have been discussing moisture, elasticity, and other factors which cause your skin to wrinkle. Actually, all these principles are directly related to dryness. Remember that dry skin is a forerunner of wrinkled skin. To reinforce everything you have just learned, please re-read chapter six, "The Inside Story . . . My Solution to Dry Skin."

As you read this book, you will understand more and more the needs of your skin. To fortify yourself so you can perform miracles in your skin . . . act on the following program.

SEVEN-STEP PROGRAM TO PREVENT WRINKLES

#1. PROPER USE OF THE COD LIVER OIL MINI-MILK-SHAKE.
SEE CHAPTER 6.

**#2. CHOOSE THE CORRECT BEVERAGES WITH MEALS.
SEE CHAPTER 14.**

what you should know about wrinkles

**#3. ELIMINATE HARMFUL LIQUIDS IN THE DIET.
SEE CHAPTER 14.**

what you should know about wrinkles

**#4. LEARN WHEN AND HOW TO DRINK LIQUIDS.
SEE CHAPTERS 11 and 14.**

what you should know about wrinkles

**#5. LEARN WHICH OILS TO KEEP AWAY FROM.
SEE CHAPTER 7.**

what you should know about wrinkles

**#6. LEARN ABOUT VITAMINS AND HOW THEY RE-
LATE TO YOUR SKIN.
SEE CHAPTER 16.**

**#7. LEARN FACTS ABOUT FOOD, PREPARATION,
MENUS, AND RECIPES FOR DRY SKIN.
SEE CHAPTER 15.**

Up to this point, we have covered the principle needs of skin—and how to fulfill them.

Now we come to grips with four baffling skin diseases.

9

The four major skin diseases ... Acne, Eczema, Psoriasis, Skin Cancer

Acne, eczema, psoriasis, and skin cancer are the four major skin diseases. There are specific individual causes for each one of these diseases.

Acne and eczema might be regarded as diseases of the young, although some afflicted souls have had to contend with these unsightly and uncomfortable lesions all their lives. Psoriasis seems not especially prone to any age group, and skin cancer, by and large, affects adults.

There are some generalities which apply to all of these diseases, and these will be summed up later in the chapter. For now, it is preferable that we address ourselves to each problem individually.

Acne

Acne is a skin infection and eruption which occurs when the sebaceous ducts become clogged, rendering the skin incapable of performing its normal secretory function. Stated simply, acne occurs when the skin is asked to handle types of oils which are metabolically unadaptable. Like most diseases, acne is a symptom of a larger constitutional disorder. These red, unsightly nodules of unusual persistence are nature's way of telling us that we are eating incorrectly.

Specifically, acne results from a continued intake of fried oils and/or oils with low metabolic activity. Hydrogenated oils (such as are found in most margarine, cheap ice creams and peanut butters) also can cause acne.

The sebaceous ducts are most vulnerable in the ten–eighteen age bracket, when the body is undergoing other great transformations. Because of this, acne is often associated with pubescence. In years past, it was often thought a boy with acne was suffering mainly from sexual frustration, and that, later, marriage would cure the problem. The truth of the matter is that these formative years present a great burden upon the developing body. It is highly vulnerable to abuse and is undergoing constant and sensitive changes. The boy is becoming a man and the girl is developing into a woman. With this unique, demanding phenomenon, the body is called upon to deal with numerous glandular pressures simultaneously. It is a period of almost constant biologic stress, and a time when it is pure folly to burden the body any further than need be. Unfortunately, our culture is such that this is also the period of life when young adults are first eating out of the home. New taste sensations are available; fast-food franchises are on every corner; money is available for just such delights. But fast-food establishments do things the easiest, cheapest way, which guarantees the use of fried oil, fried salt, and foods which are already devitalized.

One might ask, "Does acne just affect the young?" As I have stated, the most worrisome years are ten to eighteen, the reason being the young body's vulnerability. By the time the physical body has completely matured, the taste preferences and eating habits have been set to the point the body is acclimated to a certain amount of abuse. It has, in a way, developed a "tolerance" to bad dietary habits. For this reason, adults can get by without contracting acne even though they occasionally eat fried oils and fried salt.

This must not be interpreted as an endorsement of these junk foods, irrespective of age. Your body pays a price at all times. Specifically, continued use of salt—especially fried salt—predisposes one to high blood pressure, a degenerative disease many times more destructive than acne.

It is interesting to note that acne was a medical rarity fifty years ago. Also, there has been an enormous dietary change that has overcome North America in the last fifty years. But neither the American diet, nor the acne it produces, is static. As the American diet spreads around the world, so too does this skin disorder. (Ireland is an interesting but completely understandable exception among "modern" "Western" nations. The Irish diet remains basic and wholesome; therefore there is little acne in Ireland.)

But most of the rest of the world has adopted, or is adopting, the American "eat-on-the-run," "theater snacks" type of diet. The potato chip, the french fry, popcorn, and peanuts all contain fried oil plus heated salt. Salt, in any abundance, contricts the kidney arteries, so that the body's toxic wastes—rather than being normally eliminated—are forced back into the body via the blood stream, where they must then seek other outlets. These add to the aggravation caused by the prior clogging of the sebaceous gland at the opening, and infection sets in. The infection can be further spread if sugary liquids are introduced into the diet.

The most destructive addition to the American diet since World War II has been hydrogenated margarine, because it has such a low metabolic activity. When it reaches the skin, the skin can't use it; therefore, it lies there, like a puddle, like a quagmire of oil—a surface oil which becomes sebum. Considering its destructive potential and all the eventual damage it can do, it can be likened to an oil slick at sea.

Recall, high-quality oils are capable of delivering healing power to the skin, but a presence of low-quality oils hinders this process. Further, soft drinks increase the congealing of oils, so that the skin's natural healing ability is further stunted. The most vital property of the skin—its healing capacity—is thus neutralized.

If acne infections are permitted to continue, they finally become scar tissue, and later, keloids (blisters with nodule-like scars under them) and then the final scar—the inferiority complex which invariably descends upon the bearer—has been formed.

Eczema

Children can be born with eczema, and when this happens, we know it is the diet of the mother that was responsible. Usually she lays this groundwork by consuming improper liquids with meals during her pregnancy. Sometimes full-blown eczema is not apparent in the newborn; instead we see dry, sallow, ashen skin, which again points to inadequacy in the mother's diet. If, from this point, she responds by feeding the infant canned or frozen juices, the road to eczema is open.

By a similar token, if the child lives the first ten years of life without showing signs of eczema, it is unlikely that that child will ever develop it. This is because the road to eczema frequently begins with the mother's diet.

Eczema is essentially a disease stemming from unneutralized acid intake into the body. As stated earlier, if we eat an orange, this is acceptable, because we are chewing the acid, and the saliva produced neutralizes it.

But the acid in canned or frozen orange juice is drunk, and the natural neutralizing agent (saliva) is not brought into use. Orange blends are even worse. If you ask your skin to buffer the acids you should have chewed in your mouth, the skin cannot do it. Therefore, the chances are great that eczema can develop anytime we drink juices, vinegar, tea, soft drinks, etc. But even here, we are given warning signs. Before the eczema develops, we will have seen a change in our elbows from normal to whitish, to scaly, to dusty, to smoky, and finally, to a greenish hue.

The word *eczema,* according to Dr. S. L. Andelman, writing in the *Los Angeles Times*

(3/11/76), is not always used with clinical precision. Some authorities, he says, regard eczema to be "anything that looks like eczema." In any event, it is a disease with the capacity to drive one near-insane with itching. The first and most critical step in the treatment centers about diagnosis, which is not always easy. If the patient waits until the eczematous skin eruption has been present for a long time, the skin may have been treated with so many medications that its appearance may have been modified.

Whatever the case, eczema is a serious matter. It has undergone a biological "hardening" during the last several thousand years and today causes more allergy and results in greater sensitivity than ever. Chemicals have caused this. Today we are even confronted with "contact" eczema which can be brought on by wearing nylon underwear.

Today's sophisticated forms of eczema— which are real headaches—result in the main from our so-called advanced food technology, and from synthetic fabrics.

The problem of the fabrics is simple. Wear cotton or wool.

The problem with the foods should be simple, too. But ingrained eating habits are not that easy to overcome. It isn't all that easy to prohibit cola drinks from a teenager's diet, especially if we don't see that teenager for days on end.

The preventive against the contracting of

eczema must begin in infancy. Once again, the magic elixir is Cod Liver Oil. If children are given Cod Liver Oil for the first ten years of life, they will be able to avoid the ravages of eczema—and a great deal more. If, after contracting eczema, the child (or adult) immediately goes on a regimen of Cod Liver Oil, eats only those foods listed for "Normal Skin" in the Menu section of this book, and completely refrains from acid-bearing liquids, the battle against eczema will already be half-won.

Before we leave the topic of eczema, I would like to direct an important comment relative to the burgeoning growth of food-technology and the dangerous inroads it has made. Blends which imitate real fruit juices are loaded with chemicals, preservatives, stabilizers, dyes, fillers, and just about anything else that comes to mind which will sell the product, or produce it more easily, or give it a greater shelf-life. Obviously, the trend has been established and it will become much worse before it gets any better. All the more reason for all of us to be alert to the increasing dangers and pay even greater attention to what we drink.

Psoriasis

This nasty, persistent disease has been around a long time. It is mentioned in the earliest medical writings.

Esthetically, psoriasis is an eyesore. People who have it feel just as inferior as those with acne. The skin itself seems to dry out, as if rejecting all lubricants, and parts of it become silvery and almost as scaly as a fish, and these "scales" are constantly proliferating. It strikes anywhere, but the face, scalp, legs and hands seem most vulnerable. It is often hideous and usually hangs on and on. It is highly resistant to external treatments. In fact, it cannot be effectively treated from without, nor can it be really cured in any fashion. It can be minimized almost to a point of nonexistence, but this highly desired result can only be achieved from within. Again, as with acne and eczema, the secret lies with diet, and Cod Liver Oil.

Up to 10 percent of all sufferers of rheumatoid arthritis have had a concomitant psoriasis. In years past, we rarely saw psoriasis associated with osteoarthritis, but today we see a significant incidence of young rheumatoid arthritics with psoriasis. We also see a considerable amount of it among people in young and middle years, without any other disorder.

The intensity of psoriasis has increased in the past twenty-five years. It used to be a slow-forming, insidious, tenacious-type skin disorder, but now it is evolving into a fast-developing, explosive disease because of the radical changes in our liquid-intake habits.

The National Psoriasis Foundation was formed in Portland, Oregon, about ten years ago. It is dedicated to the furthering of understanding about the disease, and a commitment to find a resolution to it. Since the founding of this organization, many chapters have sprung up, and there are now units scattered over the United States.

Probably the greatest contribution toward a meaningful understanding of psoriasis has been given us by Dr. John T. Voorhees of the University of Michigan. First, he has narrowed the problem down to a biochemical explanation. Short of work done in the field of nutrition, his contributions have given us the best overall characterization of the disease. He claims psoriasis is an imbalance in the skin between the AMP (adenomonophosphate) and GMP (guano-monophosphate) cycles. AMP-GMP imbalance (or balance) is what either enhances or decreases proliferation of the psoriasis lesion (the lesion is the forerunner of the "condition"). The most profound evaluation of his work is this: if we can understand the proliferation of the psoriatic cell, we will then be on our way to understanding wild cell growth (cancer).

But Dr. Voorhees' work seems destined not to proceed beyond a certain point, because he does not couple it with a knowledge and belief in nutrition. The National Psoriasis Foundation rushed to support him, but now it seems that progress has been stalled—all this because he has not examined the dietary significance of the equation.

The question has been asked time and time again why psoriasis has "enjoyed" such a resurgence of incidence. It is, after all, more prevalent now than ever. Once again I must return to a favored old friend, Cod Liver Oil, for the explanation. First, it is demonstrable that psoriasis became newly prominent just forty years ago, and it was also about forty years ago that natural Cod Liver Oil was essentially replaced by substitutes. For all practical purposes, the use of natural Cod Liver Oil was curtailed. Fish-oil capsules as well as natural and synthetic vitamins were substituted, because natural Cod Liver Oil was not profitable, and many objected to the taste. But this was an expensive transformation, for, in the losing of Cod Liver Oil, we also lost a priceless ingredient, Arachidonic Fatty Acid. This was the essential fatty acid in Cod Liver Oil, and is the epitome of all the fatty acids, for it has the greatest ability to repair tissue lesions. We learned, the very hard way, that there is absolutely no substitute for natural Cod Liver Oil. The personal role I played in 1951 in the revitalization of natural Cod Liver Oil used in the United States still gives me a feeling of warm pride. The full story of my fight to achieve this is told in chapter twelve.

This is not to say that lack of Arachidonic Fatty Acid results in psoriasis, for it does not. But add to this the lower-quality oils we ingest and the iced drink of the common daily diet. This sets the stage for the flooding of the skin with sugar at a time when its natural protections are at lowest ebb. Bombardment of the skin with sugar and acids when it is most vulnerable gives rise to a number of dire possibilities, one of which is psoriasis.

The psoriasis sufferer, then, is being given a message by nature. The message is this: Your skin is vulnerable—you must take the best care of it you can. The psoriasis sufferer for instance can withstand exposure to the sun if he has adhered to a correct diet. That is, psoriasis and the sun can go together harmoniously if the body is properly protected with lubricating oils. There are only three such lubricating oils one should take: (1) Cod Liver Oil, (2) cold-pressed vegetable oils, and (3) the fat contained in whole milk.

Moreover, psoriasis sufferers should adhere to the "Normal Skin Diet," presented in the Menu section of this book, with emphasis on raw salads. The health drink shown in the same section is highly recommended. Above all, the psoriasis sufferer should take Cod Liver Oil twice a day for the first six months (this to build up a supply of Vitamin F). Frozen juices and soft drinks are absolutely forbidden, as are other acid-bearing liquids.

I would like to end this section by mentioning that medical science has tried, and is trying, other than dietary approaches in the search for a cure for psoriasis. In fact, some of these regimens are actually palliative. Massachusetts General Hospital, in 1974, tried a combination of Egyptian reed (reduced into capsule form) and a special ultraviolet light, with some degree of success. These tests continue.

But such external remedies are doomed to fall short of their intended goal. Psoriasis, like acne and eczema, are internal disorders which are simply manifest in the condition of the skin. Until something is done to correct the basic flaw—the internal flaw—psoriasis will continue, and only temporarily yield to balms and lotions and other salutory measures. Like the housewife who sweeps dirt under the rug, no permanent improvement has been achieved.

Skin Cancer

Admittedly, there are many forms of skin cancer, ranging from the rodent ulcer, to melanoma, to epithelioma. We address ourselves here to most common forms, such as epithelioma, which are related to skin-protection-breakdown, combined with some abnormal irritant.

It is no fluke of nature that Australians have the highest incidence of skin cancer in the world. The two most deleterious components possible are common to them: a blistering Tropic-of-Capricorn sun and a great thirst for tea. Not only do Australians drink tea, but they drink the most potent Ceylonese teas they can find, and in huge amounts of it—twenty to thirty cups a day is not uncommon. Their intake of tannic acid is enormous, preparing for the loss of skin elasticity.

Skin cancer is caused when (1) the skin's defenses have been stripped, and (2) the irritant has been added. The irritant, most often, is the sun.

Stripping the skin's defenses occurs when:

(1) Iodine is leeched from the skin by drinking sugary liquids, and when
(2) The skin is supersensitized by the intake of phosphoric, tartaric (soft drinks), citric (frozen juices), or tannic (tea) acids.

A similar situation to that in Australia might be developing in some of our own southern states, especially Texas and Florida, and especially now that tennis has become so popular. Iced tea, soft drinks, etc. are all quite tempting after a grueling match on the courts. Such vicious combinations, of course, must be avoided. More, tennis players must become used to the habit of protecting their skin from excessive sunlight.

We might mention here that another great tea-drinking country, Canada, does not have an unusually high rate of skin cancer, but then, neither does it have a blistering, tropical sun.

Again, Cod Liver Oil is the greatest and most reliable protector. It goes a great distance toward replacing what has been lost. Remember, if nothing else, this one adage: "One must earn the right to sit in the sun."

Biological Individuality and the Four Skin Diseases

Some magnificent research has been done by Roger Williams, Ph.D., of the University of Texas. He contends that each of us is born with a biochemical individuality. Our bodies are as biochemically different as our fingerprints. Dr. Williams further contends that each of us has much in common—within our individualities— at birth, but that as we are subjected to the patterns of our home, we develop highly specialized eating habits. These determine, at a very early age, what diseases will later strike us. Sometimes these eating habits will quickly set the stage for disease—as in the case of eczema, which may be as little as one year in development. Other diseases, directly related to eating habits, may take twenty years to become manifest.

This is why one person will contract acne while another will be more sensitive to psoriasis, etc. The extent of our bad habits can influence the direction and seriousness of the skin disorder which may strike.

Fight Back with Nutrition

All the diseases talked about in this chapter can be overcome with a carefully designed program. They can respond favorably to:

1. The "Normal Skin" menus in chapter fifteen.
2. The Cod Liver Oil mixture, taken properly.
3. The adherence of correctly consuming liquids.
4. Carefully noting and correcting any critical points reviewed about each disease.
5. Above all, faithful diligence to the program must be employed. Give it time. It can work wonders.

In the following chapter, I shall discuss skin problems which may or may not be illusory.

10.

Can skin problems be psychosomatic?

How many times have you heard the expression, "mind over matter"?

Psychology, the study of the mind, was introduced to the world in the latter part of the nineteenth century. Sigmund Freud, an Austrian physician, was the "father" of this science. He was followed by a long list of distinguished psychiatrists and psychoanalysts, among whom were Carl Gustav Jung, Alfred Adler, Theodore Reik, and Carl Rogers.

Many theories emerged and are still developing. But all these theorists agree that psychology can help patients understand themselves. This is most often accomplished by examining repressed feelings such as anger and guilt.

Psychosomatic means "mind" plus "body." It refers to maladies or problems that are of emotional origin. Some psychiatrists and psychologists believe disease, including skin disorder, can be triggered by anxiety and stress.

Where Does It All Begin?

I believe rashes and some serious skin disease can result from psychological origins. But I pose this question, "Which came first, the sick mind or the sick body?"

When the body is denied specific nutrients the skin needs, you can almost be certain the brain is also being shortchanged.

Genetics—The Blueprint of the Body

The laws of genetics establish individual characteristics for each of us. This applies to every area of the body, including the skin. No two people's blueprints are exactly the same. But regardless of your personal biology—whether you have oily, dry-oily, or wrinkled skin—the information in these pages can help you understand your individual needs.

Skin—The Mirror of Our Feelings

All of us have seen how skin reflects the mind's anxieties. During times of fear, the skin can take on an ashen pallor. Embarrassment produces flushing. "Goose bumps" or perspiration can be responses to fear or sensuality.

Fortunately, these skin flare-ups are of short duration. Flare-ups are one of the ways by which we give vent to strong emotional feelings. We are simply "blowing off steam."

Serious Skin Disorders Can Change Our Lives

While it is debatable that emotional disorders can cause skin problems, there is no question that the reverse is true. Skin afflictions can make life miserable.

Acne, psoriasis, eczema, vitiligo and even skin cancer are nutrition-related skin disorders which cling stubbornly and usually grow worse. Aside from discomfort and loss of skin vitality, these disorders also have the effect of making one feel socially inferior. Confidence in one's appearance is lost, and such a loss is sometimes difficult to overcome completely, even after restoration of skin health.

Vitamin Megadosage

Today we see break-throughs in the treatment of psychological problems. Vitamins are playing a role in these innovative treatments.

The theory is that many mental functions depend upon a good chemical balance in the body. For example, some forms of depression are relieved by upgraded nutrition. Vitamins play a role in the establishment of nutritional balance. As with any other machine, the whole of the human body cannot work unless the parts are functioning properly. And, as with those other machines, proper functioning only results from care and attention.

The biochemistry of the body is such that we must always regard it as one interrelated unit. When there are deficiencies, the biochemistry is thrown out of balance. This can cause hazardous results to the mind, to the skin, on throughout the body. One recent break-through of great importance has been in the field of vitamin megadosage. Dr. Abram Hoffer, a Canadian psychiatrist, of Victoria, British Columbia has treated his patients with huge doses of vitamins. In *Nutrition and Your Mind*, Dr. George Watson makes an excellent argument to show a direct connection between nutritional intake and the healthy mind.

The work of Drs. Hoffer and Watson has taken us forward by leaps and bounds, and really does address the crux of the matter. I believe that while it is important to be able to ply the body with vitamins, this does not do enough toward good assimilation of the vitamins already present in our diets. Furthermore, I believe recovery would be accelerated if these megadosages were more properly administered. Taken with water, as is so often the case, their efficiency is greatly diminished. Among the common vitamins taken, A, D, E, and K are oil soluble and therefore should be taken only with oil-bearing liquids.

Life Is Better When You Know the Rules

No one is exempt from emotional stress, tragedy, or trauma. I highly respect the insights afforded us by the science of psychology. In no way is there a conflict between the teachings of psychology and the teachings of nutrition. The two sciences, in fact, enhance one another.

If you keep fit and are attentive to nutrition, you will be better able to deal with the realities of life. And you will not then be the victim of a so-called psychosomatic affliction.

Questions and Answers

In this section of the book we have set forth our belief that psychosomatic illness is much more fancy than fact.

To more fully demonstrate this, I offer the

following questions—which have come to me over
the years—and their corresponding answers.

Q. I have been told by my dermatologist that my skin condition
—Called vitiligo—is based on my psychological feelings? Do
you think that's true?

A. I do not. Vitiligo occurs when there is a serious shortage of
the B vitamins in the body. Sometimes it can be genetic; it
can also result from glandular exhaustion.

Q. I have itchiness and scaliness around my nose, eyebrows and
hairline. My psychiatrist tells me this is happening because
of nervousness. Is this true?

A. I disagree. As I have outlined throughout this book, scaliness and dandruff of the skin and scalp are the result of
incorrect eating and drinking.

Q. I have shingles right now. I have been told that it's because
I am going through a divorce, that it's all just a case of
nerves. Can this be so?

A. *Herpes Zoster* is commonly called shingles. Have you ever
considered how many people are getting divorced these days
—and who thus have great stress in their lives—who do not
get shingles? If your body is fortified with enough lubrication and B vitamins (protection against stress), you need not
get shingles. You set the stage for such skin outbreaks as
Herpes Zoster by drinking frozen juices, carbonated drinks,
etc. It is just part of the cause—as I have said throughout
the book.

Q. I have had *Acne Rosacea* for years. My skin doctor has not
been able to help me. He suggests it may be psychological.
Is that possible?

A. *Acne Rosacea* is a very long-term, chronic skin disorder affecting the skin of the nose, forehead, and cheeks, as is
marked by flushing and followed by red coloration caused
by dilation of the capillaries. As a rule, it is the result of a
lengthy history of dietary blunders and nutritional mistakes.

Q. I have some relatives in Alabama whose children have pellagra. One is mentally retarded. What brought this on? Is
there a direct relationship between the two disorders?

A. Pellagra is an endemic skin and spinal disease most common to Southern Europe and the south and central parts of
the United States. It is caused by a deficiency of nicotinic
acid and can become a serious ailment, indeed, with end
results affecting both the spinal column and the brain. Crippling and idiocy are known to occur. But despite the dire

seriousness of the disorder, it can be quickly cured if caught in time. There is no reason to believe it is caused by emotional problems.

Q. I have an extensive redness on both sides of my neck. It has been with me for years and there seems to be no effective remedy for it. Do you have any idea what this might be, and if it can be alleviated?

A. It sounds suspiciously like *neurodermatitis*. This is generally caused when the kidneys are not operating well. The sweating on the neck produces toxic materials which inflame the skin. The best antidote I know would be a moss-extract solution swabbed on the neck daily after showering. But the diet also has to be corrected so as to increase the function of the kidneys. Incidentally, I call this condition the "Redneck."

Next we come to a subject that has been misrepresented. Cholesterol, even today, is very much a source of confusion to many people.

Reading the next chapter will clarify this subject.

Part Three

THE OVERLOOKED NEEDS OF THE SKIN

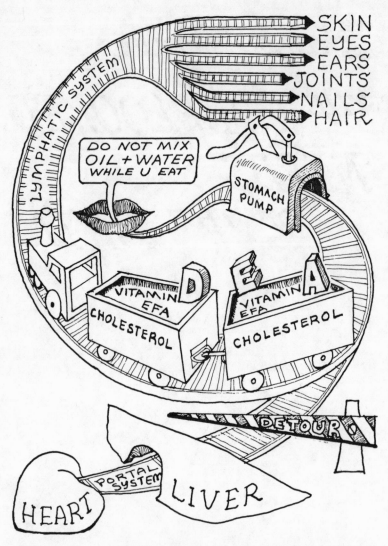

Selected dietary oils are
necessary for your skin.
The trick is —
learn how to assimilate
them to avoid harm.

11

Cholesterol and your skin

Cholesterol is a natural product of the skin. The amount and quality of cholesterol in the skin determines its health and youthfulness. This substance is vitally necessary to transport oil-soluble Vitamin A and essential fatty acids throughout your body . . . in order to maintain proper lubrication.

What is cholesterol? It is a fat-like, pearly substance found in animal fats and oils, in bile, blood, brain tissue, milk, yolk of egg, the liver, the medullated sheaths of fibers, kidneys, and adrenal glands.

Unfortunately, too often the benefits of cholesterol never reach the skin because cholesterol takes a wrong turn. It usually winds up in the arteries of the heart or in some other vascular tissue.

In this chapter I tell <u>why</u> this happens and you will see that it is <u>not</u> due to the consumption of cholesterol-bearing foods.

My dietary techniques are designed to promote a stable and normal level of cholesterol in your blood stream.

I want to go on record to say that cholesterol has been greatly misunderstood. Too much misleading information has been spread about the dangers of cholesterol as it relates to heart disease. These statements have been made without sufficient scientific corroboration.

Important Research on Cholesterol

We are fortunate in having some medical doctors with open and probing minds. They have observed this "cholesterol problem" through long-term medical studies. The following data are but a small part of research that questions the validity of the accepted myths about cholesterol.

Dr. Paul Dudley White, the renowned American heart specialist and former physician to President Dwight D. Eisenhower, was correct when he said the following: "I think I have a pretty clear idea of the role of proteins, carbohydrates and so forth, but I must admit I'm not sure whether some form of the weight control diets might not be dan-

gerous to the heart. The amount in the blood—
we call it plasma cholesterol—is <u>not</u> necessarily
related to the cholesterol found in food."

Dr. George V. Mann, professor of biochemistry and medicine at Vanderbilt University, was
even more definitive. He called the entire hypothesis of altering the kinds of fat, in order to
reduce heart disease, as being over-promoted and
over-publicized.

This physician went on to say: "The theory
that fatty acid metabolism plays a role in heart disease is a 'myth' that has been a terribly wasteful
diversion for the medical community. After twenty
years and several hundred million dollars, we still
do not see any convincing evidence in its support."

During the late fifties a well-known medical
research project was started. It was the Framingham Study, directed by Dr. William B. Kannel.
He hoped to uncover cholesterol's relationship to
heart attacks.

Dr. Kannel stated that a blood test for cholesterol was probably the most useful measure to
show existing or even impending heart disease.
Thousands of men and women in the city of Framingham, Massachusetts, were then examined. In
this project doctors tried to relate heart disease to
any and all known theoretical causes.

After fourteen years all that was discovered
was that half of the people in the study (who died

of heart attacks) had no prior laboratory evidence of elevated blood cholesterol. It can be said the blood test for cholesterol is useful, but certainly not fully conclusive.

Furthermore, Dr. Kannel determined that there was no relationship between what a person ate and the level of his blood cholesterol.

Here I strongly differ with Dr. Kannel's assumption. I <u>know</u> that a proper diet is an <u>important part</u>, even though only a part of the answer, that will deter heart disease.

Similar experiments, such as the Framingham Study, were conducted in New York City, Seattle, and in England. They all reported more or less the same results.

Jeopardy to Our Infants

There is a further consequence of great danger to our very young, if the misconception about cholesterol continues.

Pediatricians are now beginning to suggest that young mothers feed their babies nonfat milk. Dr. Peter O. Kwiterovich, a pediatrician at John Hopkins University School of Medicine, says: "No one really knows how brain growth would be affected if a child were to receive a low cholesterol diet before he is 24 months of age, at which time 95 percent of brain growth is completed."

I believe, since there has been no clear-cut substantiation of this theory, that it is unwise to jeopardize our infants.

Some Current Reports on Cholesterol

In the *Los Angeles Times* (June 20, 1974) there was a column by Professor Jean Mayer, then professor of Nutrition at Harvard University. His article was entitled "Some Diets Hazardous to Health." Cholesterol was the main subject of the article.

He discussed a careful study at the Cardiovascular Laboratory, Department of Medicine at the Peter Bent Brigham Hospital and the Harvard Medical School. He clearly stated that the low carbohydrate and high protein diets recommended by Doctors Irwin M. Stillman and Robert Atkins are dangerous to your health.

Other doctors reported their findings in an article published in the *Journal of the American Medical Association*. They also evaluated Dr. Stillman's book quite unfavorably.

The *Los Angeles Times* pointed out that these diets mainly consist of eating unlimited quantities of lean beef, veal, or lamb with the visible fat trimmed off, chicken and turkey with the skin removed, flounder, cod, haddock, etc. Needless to say, this is a high protein diet. Little mention was made of the fact that this diet also happens to be high in saturated fat and cholesterol.

This was a short-term experiment of weeks. As long as the patients stayed on the diet, their blood cholesterol level steadily increased from an average of 215 milligrams per 100 milliliters to 248 milligrams per 100 milliliters when they quit. The authors reported that if such a rapid elevation of some 15 percent were to persist, it would induce a sizable hike in the risk of coronaries or strokes.

Dr. Stillman stressed that the diet should include at least eight glasses of water every day, as well as quantities of low calorie beverages.

Here is where Dr. Stillman's diet became dangerous in my judgment.

This applies to Dr. Atkins' diet as well, which allows the oil-free liquids such as skim milk, coffee, tea, and diet sodas with meals.

In the book, *The Cholesterol Controversy* by Dr. Edward Pinckney and his wife Cathey, published in 1973, is the story of the Somali and Masai tribes of Tanganyika. Both tribes drink enormous amounts of milk and are heavy meat eaters. The milk drunk by them—up to five quarts a day—has been found to have twice the amount of fat content of the milk used on the American table.

Both tribes have an average blood cholesterol level of 125 mg. to 150 mg. percent. In contrast to our normal range in this part of the world of 150 mg. to 250 mg. percent, I found this to be interesting. They consume much fatty meat and rich milk, supposedly a sure way of producing high cholesterol counts.

In the same vein, the Seventh Day Adventists have some 70 percent less heart disease and 30 percent less cancer. They are lacto-ova-vegetarians. They drink milk, eat eggs and vegetables, as well as fruits and cheese. They do not drink coffee or tannic acid teas.

The United States government is projecting further research about why Seventh Day Adventists have this phenomenal good health.

My Own Analysis of the Cholesterol Problem

Since the 1940s the average American was counseled by his doctor to avoid many cholesterol-bearing foods. We were told to swing to polyunsaturates. Millions of people took the route to polyunsaturates.

Then came "big business" with similar high pressure advertising campaigns. Margarine was championed to take over the role of butter. We were also urged to use low-fat dairy products.

In spite of all this medically-inspired caution, heart disease has actually skyrocketed. The emphasis on unsaturated fats was ill-advised.

Simultaneously, we deprived our skin of essential oils.

Skin and Heart Problems Showing up in Youths

In my research I have observed great changes in the skin of young people since World War II. Extremes of both dry and oily skin are more apparent. There is no doubt in my mind that diet changes have had a big effect.

Until the age of twelve or thirteen, the liquids consumed with meals are usually whole milk or soup. Then soft drinks, frozen juices, ice water, and similar liquids free of any oil are frequently substituted.

The big switch in liquids interferes with good assimilation and creates serious changes in the body, including your cholesterol.

There were some shocking reports that came out in the Korean War records. In autopsies of young American soldiers, eighteen through twenty-one years of age, it was found that their arteries were like those found in men from eighty to ninety years of age.

Certainly these arteries did not harden on the battlefields in a few months.

Assimilation, unfortunately, is not understood or reviewed sufficiently. It is so important to your skin I will discuss it now.

Assimilation—Where Cholesterol Becomes Friend or Foe; How to Feed Your Skin Without Harming Your Heart

One serious problem, as I have said in this book, is the oil crisis in most of our bodies. This could happen because of a variety of reasons.

The oils in our food may be inferior or inadequate. Also, it could be that the oils and fats in the diet are being diverted from the systemic (lymphatic) system. It is through this systemic pipe line that our bodies are lubricated.

It is when improper assimilation occurs that the oils are led away from our lubricating route. Assimilation, starting in the stomach, sets in motion the direction and performance of cholesterol.

For years doctors have classified the stomach as a vessel. You should also remember that it is a pumping vessel. It has two openings. One is the esophagus tube through which your food enters, the other is the pyloric valve through which the food passes into the intestinal tract.

The purpose of the stomach is to digest solid foods and liquify fats. Most food changes into a homogenous mixture called chyme. However, fat is merely liquified into an oil by the heat in the stomach. Neither fat nor oil is ever digested there. It is merely pumped by the stomach to either the

portal system (through the liver) or the systemic
route (around the liver). Medically, it is known
as the lymphatic system.

There is a simple fact of life that you must
look at. It governs the quality of your assimilation.
OIL AND WATER DO NOT MIX. This
law was proven in a vessel. No matter how long
the attempt to blend these two substances, they do
not mix. You would not combine water and oil
together in the oil or water pump of your car.

The same principle applies to the human
body. Why the people of the world have been combining oil-free liquids (water, coffee, tea, soft
drinks, frozen juices, beer, whiskey, wine, and
skim milk) with oil-bearing foods in the stomach
. . . just does not make good sense.

When you break a law what happens? You
pay a penalty. The penalty in this case is . . .
cholesterol winding up in the arteries of the heart
instead of being properly metabolized in your
skin.

Usually, it requires an average of four hours
or more for a meal to be digested. To assure good
assimilation you should consume an oil-bearing
liquid (whole milk or homemade soup) with your
meal.

Why have I suggested that you drink milk
(which is 87 percent water) with your oil-bearing
food? The liquid in milk is water of low surface

tension. This low-surface-tension liquid does blend with oil or fat. Plain water and most all oil-free liquids are of a high surface tension. They do not blend with oil.

Whole milk that is not homogenized has the cream on the top and thin watery milk below.

When milk is homogenized, thoroughly shaken, it becomes blended and the cream is broken down into tiny fat globules. All fats from your food must be broken into tiny globules before they can be properly assimilated.

At mealtime it is your choice of the correct liquid that will make possible good assimilation. When this occurs, about 70 to 80 percent of the dietary oils and fats will then go around your liver. The essential oils will now be able to pass on to other parts of your body—where lubrication, moisturization, and healing are needed. This can be the protection for a healthy skin as well as a healthy heart.

How Do the Oils Become Beneficial . . . or Harmful?

At the end of your digestive tract there is actually a divided vascular highway. The left portion is the portal circulatory branch. This route is through the liver, eventually leading to the arteries and on to the heart. The right side is the systemic circulatory channel. It will propel oil into the peripheral circulation to feed the skin and other parts of the body.

Here is an example of how the oils wind up going through the portal branch, the liver:

Let us say that you are having a meal and with it you are having coffee, or you may have the coffee right after your meal. You are committing the act of combining oil (from your meal) with water (from your coffee). What happens? Instead of the liquid blending with the solid food, the liquid and the fat in the food are at odds—they separate. When this occurs, the combining of the liquid that is not compatible with the fat in the food causes puddling of the oils. This is called coalescing.

Coalescing causes a chain action with an added strain being put on the gall bladder and the pancreas. The job of the gall bladder is to produce bile salts to emulsify the fats in your diet. Emulsifying breaks down the larger coalesced globules to the required small size.

After the gall bladder performs its task, the pancreas has to take over. It secretes a fat-splitting enzyme called lipase. This enzyme breaks down the emulsified globules into fatty acids. Now the oil is ready for assimilation.

This all takes place in the portal system on its way to the liver . . . away from the skin.

First, I want you to understand more about the liver. The liver is the largest internal organ of the body and acts as a chemical plant. The liver synthesizes proteins, processes carbohydrates, absorbs fat products, and makes them available as fuel.

It also serves as a storehouse for vitamins and minerals, processes iron for the blood system, and renders harmless some of the poisons that enter your blood stream. You can see that its primary function is the conversion of digested food coming from the digestive tube.

When the majority of the oils in your food is shunted through the portal system, the liver is the greatest benefactor. The oil-soluble vitamins and essential fatty acids are extrapolated there and stored. Very little gets out to the rest of the body.

If the liver metabolizes all the oils, then they burn as fuel. This burning process is chemically known as desaturation.

It is my belief that this desaturation process results in the production of cholesterol crystals. One result could be the showering of your heart muscle with deposits of cholesterol.

So you can see that if you continue to mix oil and water in your stomach, you will also injure your gall bladder and pancreas. You will strain and overwork these two organs meal after meal.

They (the cholesterol crystals) can then go on to deposit themselves along the walls of the

arteries throughout your body. This eventually
causes both narrowing and hardening of the arteries. At this point after a physical, your doctor may
find that you have high blood pressure, arteriosclerosis, and poor circulation.

Unfortunately, the process of proper assimilation is not widely understood. Because of this,
countless people are suffering from a lack of precious oil-soluble vitamins and essential fatty acids
needed to feed specific areas of the body. This is
largely owing to poor distribution, initially caused
by improper assimilation.

Cholesterol Can Be Your Skin's Best Friend

Cholesterol, acquired through your food, is
beneficial if assimilated well. It is found in milk,
butter, eggs, cheese, meat, fish, etc. This type of
edible cholesterol is known as exogenous. To be
beneficial it must merge with the existing endoge-
nous cholesterol already in the blood stream.

Today the natural balance of food is changing. It is being fractured or fractionated. Even the
fat from milk and cheese is being removed. Eggs,
too, are being altered. Some poultry farms are at-
tempting to produce eggs with a low cholesterol
content.

More "fractured foods" keep appearing on

the market all the time. One of the worst examples is margarine, which is cholesterol-free. It has been plasticized with the aid of nickel. It pollutes the human body and your system cannot properly metabolize it.

I have revealed in this chapter the importance of cholesterol to your skin. Another big key that is sadly lacking in many lives is the story of assimilation. Often, when one becomes ill after living on a so-called balanced diet, it may be hard to understand why. The meals become unbalanced when an incompatible liquid is consumed at the same time as the solid food.

Assimilation is not taught in our educational school system or in our medical schools. I feel, simply, that it has been overlooked. The importance of this cannot be stressed strongly enough.

In the next chapter you will find another one of your skin's best friends.

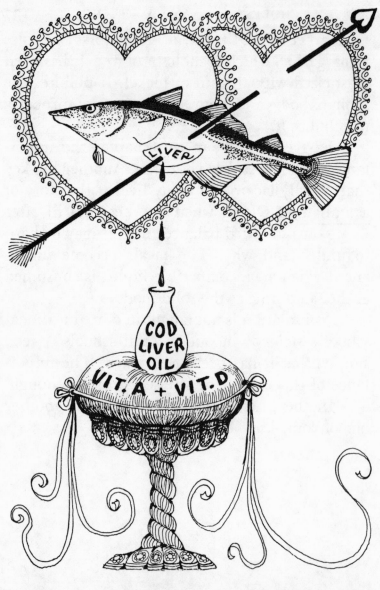

The almost mystical powers of cod liver oil

12.

My romance with cod liver oil

The almost mystical powers of Cod Liver Oil for a supple, healthy skin was revealed to me early in life. It came about in an unexpected way. Since then I have had what might be called a romance with Cod Liver Oil.

I speak of it in my lectures. I talk about it on TV and radio, and it is always included in my writings. They say that I am the greatest champion of this fantastic oil in history. Maybe so, even I smile when newspaper writers call me, "THE COD-FATHER."

How My Romance Began

It all happened because my mother was agonized with rheumatism (now referred to as arthritis). Trying to get relief, she had faithfully followed counsel from her doctors. She took pain pills, applied heat, and finally had all her teeth removed. All to no avail. Because of these failures I became agitated enough to see if perhaps I could find some relief for her.

At the beginning of my search, I stumbled onto a book in the waiting room of my dentist's office. Among the reading matter there lay a book . . . *Dorland's Medical Dictionary.*

When I came to the word "rickets" (shortly after the word "rheumatism"), I read that Cod Liver Oil was considered as a cure. That planted a seed in my mind for bones, joints, and rheumatism.

Later I read about some research that Dr. L. Duncan Bulkley, a famous dermatologist, had conducted. He had written of the wonderful effects of slightly warm milk when consumed on an empty stomach. The very young children that followed this routine acquired rosy cheeks and abundant good health.

I thought about the combination of the milk and the Cod Liver Oil. It seemed like a good idea for health and rheumatism, as well as an improvement in the taste of the Cod Liver Oil.

My mother was willing to try it. We were hoping and praying it would cause the pain to disappear—for her rheumatism to leave.

The Hidden Power of Cod Liver Oil

What developed was unexpected and surprising.

After taking the oil regularly each morning on an empty stomach, my mother noticed a series of curious changes. The first happened after ten weeks passed.

Her hair, which had been lifeless and dry, had its lustre and sheen back. Two weeks later, her skin that had been very dry, had become soft and supple. Next, she felt a sensation in her ears, and found some earwax. For several years prior, she had not evidenced any earwax at all.

The last noticeable change was what she had hoped for in the beginning: In the twenty-second week the pain left her joints.

I was astounded by all this. I realized at that time something about the anatomy I had not heard of, and have not to this day. Our bodies need lubrication to run smoothly. Even as a piece of machinery, it needs oil not to get dried out and rusty. It was a mystery to me that, heretofore, no one had found that the oiling of the body had to be done from within.

Friends of my mother tried the same technique successfully. As the word spread, and with all the happy results, I was inspired to write my first book, *Arthritis and Common Sense*.

This dramatic event became the turning point in my life. A wealth of information and experience have been revealed to me since.

My dedication to Cod Liver Oil is complete. To document my firm conviction, and to provide medical proof, let's go back about two hundred years.

The History—and Mystery—of Cod Liver Oil

Early in the eighteenth century, fishermen along the Scottish and English coasts began to tell each other how Cod Liver Oil was helping to relieve joint pain. (Commonly called rheumatism, at that time.) Similar reports came from fishing communities in Scandinavia.

The Laplanders and the Greenlanders are known to have eaten Cod Liver Oil. It was also used as a remedy for rickets and tuberculosis.

These stories eventually came to the attention of doctors. They began trying it on their patients.

Dr. Ludovicus Josephus de Jongh, of The Hague, Netherlands, did some extensive work with Cod Liver Oil. He wrote some papers in 1842 reporting how he successfully used it in his medical practice.

He stated: *After the excellent results obtained by the use of Cod Liver Oil in the various scrofulous complaints I had under my treatment in the course of the year 1842, I have reason to consider Cod Liver Oil as a curative.*

(*Scrofula* is the ancient medical term for tuberculosis. Scrofula, a widespread disease at that time, settled in many areas of the body. In the lymph nodes, in the bones, lungs, and even in parts of the stomach.)

Later, Dr. de Jongh wrote in a publication entitled <u>Lancet</u>: *In my experience in the use of Cod Liver Oil, which extends over a period of twelve years, I have never seen any ill consequence result nor has any been noticed by the different authors who have written on the subject. On the contrary, it has seldom failed, when long persevered in, to afford amelioration of the symptoms in those cases where a cure could not be effected. It may be given with confidence in all cases where the powers of life are low, and where the improper assimilation of the food is the cause. It affords nourishment when none can be borne, restores the functions of digestion, and furnishes the frame with fat in a truly wonderful manner.*

This pioneering physician, de Jongh, gave case histories. Among the maladies upon which he used Cod Liver Oil successfully were:

Chronic Rheumatism
Sciatica
Hemicrany
Cardialgia
Rheumatic Tic Douloureux
Chronic Gout
Rheumatic and Gouty Palsy
Scrofulous Diathesis
Tumefaction of the Lymphatic
  Glands
Scrofulous Ulcers
Chronic Exanthemata

Scrofulous Ophthalmia
Infantine Atrophy
Rachitis
Osteomalaxy
Scrofulous Caries
Scrofulous Affections of the
  Joints
Tubercular Consumption and
  Divers
Disturbances in the functions
  of the system of the Mucous
  Membranes

What properties are contained in Cod Liver Oil which make this substance so effective? Give full credit to Dr. de Jongh, because he took a chemical analysis of Cod Liver Oil. He found the following ingredients:

Oleic Acid, Margaric Acid, Glycerine, Butyric Acid, Acetic Acid, Fellinic Acid, Sulphuric Acid, Phosphorus, Chalk, Chalinic Acid, Bilfellinic Acid, Bilifulvine, Iodine, Bromine and Chlorine, Phosphoric Acid, Magnesia, Soda.

We now know that the above list of ingredients should also have included important vitamins . . . but vitamins were not discovered until the 1920s. Then, years later, additional essential fatty acids were identified. One of the most valuable, arachidonic, was among them.

(What he may not have realized—and one advantage which I consider important—is that the liver of any animal or mammal is where the best nutritional reserves are stored.)

Cod Liver Oil was highly appreciated for its versatility in the healing of so many ailments. This was in spite of the fact its taste was extremely unpleasant in its early form. The liver was left to rot in a barrel, then the oil was skimmed from the top.

About 1853, the steam process was introduced by Muller, and the quality and the taste improved. The popularity of Cod Liver Oil grew so that the demand was soon a pawn in the hands of the suppliers. Some tampering began to occur. Decayed herring oil and seal fat were added to it . . . making it vicious tasting. More serious than that, it became inefficient in its healing qualities.

Dr. de Jongh observed that, at times, some of the oil was ineffective. He was determined to learn why this happened. He tracked down the evidence of the adulteration that was causing it to be impure and inferior.

Through his perseverance he made pure Cod Liver Oil available. His findings also indicated that the best cod came from the coldest waters around Norway. The warmer waters did not have cuttlefish, which is an important part of the healthier codfish's diet. (This is why I have always advocated Norwegian Cod Liver Oil.)

Dr. de Jongh's dedication to bringing pure Cod Liver Oil to the people did not go unnoticed. He was honored by Her Majesty, The queen of Netherlands, for bringing such a simple and miraculous remedy to the rich and poor alike. Later he was further commended by Dr. Fouquier, professor at the University of Paris and physician to His Majesty, Louis Phillippe, king of France.

The merits of Cod Liver Oil began appearing in medical textbooks. Drs. Henoch (1882), Meiggs and Repper (1886), Starr (1894), Holt (1896), Kerly (1907), and Fischer (1907), all recommended the use of Cod Liver Oil.

Experiments in the late 1880s with dog and farm animals stricken with rickets were conclusive that Cod Liver Oil was a cure.

In 1913, Vitamin A was recognized by Mendel and McCollum. Cod Liver Oil was found to be rich in this factor. Later, Professor McCollum found that Cod Liver Oil was also rich in Vitamin D.

Dr. Chick (1923), in Vienna, found that Cod Liver Oil was a specific in the treatment of rickets among the children there.

America Begins Its Research After World War I

One of the first reports on work being done with Cod Liver Oil appeared in the *Archives of Internal Medicine,* March, 1920. Dr. Ralph Pemberton, professor at the University of Pennsylvania and a staff member at the Abington Memo-

rial Hospital, wrote of the success in the use of
Cod Liver Oil with 400 military patients who had
arthritis. In his book called *The Medical Manage-
ment of Arthritis,* he documents this.

A historical treatise on Cod Liver Oil as a
remedy was published August, 1923, in the *American Journal of Diseases of Children.* Dr. Ruth A.
Guy, Department of Pediatrics, Yale University,
School of Medicine, presented this work. It is still
a landmark thesis, stating the therapeutic value of
this fish-liver oil.

Dr. Guy wrote of the achievements in the use
of Cod Liver Oil with chronic rheumatism, gout,
and other joint diseases, such as rickets and osteo-
malacia.

In 1963 an important discovery was published in *The Journal of the American Geriatric
Society.* Dr. Charles Ancona, director of medicine
at St. Clare's Hospital, New York City, submitted
an article on the effect of Cod Liver Oil on cholesterol. He wrote that Cod Liver Oil has a cho-
lesterol-reducing action greater than any vegetable
oil. He stated it was one of the finest cholesterol
depressants.

Perhaps the foregoing history of the many
medical men who recognized Cod Liver Oil as a
useful tool has impressed you to some extent. I
would merely like to add that since the days of
Dr. de Jongh, we have found an even greater list

of illnesses which can be ameliorated by this oil.

Scores of papers have been written and recorded in the *Index Medicus*. They report that Cod Liver Oil can also be useful in alleviating the following:

Eczema	Bronchitis	Intestinal disorders
Psoriasis	Acne	High blood pressure
Pruritus	Impetigo	Anticoagulant effects
Anemia	Ulcers	Common cold
Reproductivity	Cysts	Retinitis
Menstrual	Lupus (DLE)	Cornea opacity
regulation	Breast	Night blindness
Dental caries	inflammation	Emphysema
Burns, wounds	Varicose veins	

Practical Reasons Why Cod Liver Oil Is Effective

Cod Liver Oil has essential fatty acids. Especially arachidonic. Medical science has yet to learn about the fantastic healing power of this special fatty acid.

Cod Liver Oil has iodine. It can act as a bacterial agent . . . killing certain bacteria.

Cod Liver Oil has phosphorus. This is important for tissue repair.

Cod Liver Oil helps in the natural production of body cortisone and most of the sex hormones. This happens when the Vitamin D in the oil physiologically activates the cortex of the adrenal gland.

What I have covered mostly in this chapter,

so far, is that Cod Liver Oil has wonderful healing qualities.

It was made clear to me that it has much more than healing qualities. Namely, that it is a lubricant. It achieves still another magic. Moisturization. For thousands of years we have been looking for this elusive ingredient for the skin.

I believe my unique method in the way to take Cod Liver Oil created a magic formula. The proper blending with milk did the trick. The unusual technique promoted the fullest potential of this miraculous fish oil.

The Mystery Behind the Rise and Fall of Cod Liver Oil

Yes, it is puzzling why Cod Liver Oil hasn't had more acceptance. It is especially baffling after seeing its amazing history of accomplishment against suffering and disease.

I say its taste has been the prime reason for its disfavor.

Cod Liver Oil . . . A Miracle Benefit Almost Lost

It is apparent to me that, because of the absence of greater medical interest, the merits of

Cod Liver Oil are an important loss to humanity. This has happened in spite of the fine work achieved by the resourceful medical pioneers who have used Cod Liver Oil.

The majority of doctors, working under the influence of the microbial theory (treating illness after it is formed—by drugs) seldom take time to search for preventive measures. Fortunately, for humanity's sake, there were and are exceptions.

I have already cited the critical work of Dr. Charles Ancona of St. Clare's Hospital, New York City. With our concern over cholesterol problems, he made an outstanding contribution, but it did not excite the medical world. Doctors failed to look into the value of this work. Patients across the world never got the benefit of this finding. His work rests in the medical journal, unappreciated.

Instead, margarine is still advised as an aid in reducing cholesterol. This, of course, is a vegetable oil. Large numbers of doctors have still not found out the truth about margarine. In a later chapter, I clearly state what you should know about margarine.

Doctors who seek ways of preventing illness through natural nutrients are often ignored and even ostracized. This resistance holds back progress, and at great odds.

Digitalis is an example. It was first used by the people suffering from angina pectoris, who found this miraculous ingredient in the foxglove plant. A doctor learned of this from an old woman. Fortunately, this did get acceptance from the medical world.

Your Skin . . . Your Bones . . . Your Whole Body Needs Cod Liver Oil

We are having a new kind of epidemic in the twentieth century. We see young people on the ski slopes and other sporting fields, with a rash of broken bones—especially on the football fields.

We see senior citizens with osteoporosis. They wind up with broken hips, much too easily after any slight fall.

Bones are made predominantly of calcium and phosphorus. These two minerals are under the regulation of Vitamin D, especially oil-soluble Vitamin D, the kind found in Cod Liver Oil.

What I am saying to you is that we need Cod Liver Oil all our lives. We need to take it on a regular schedule, once a week, as long as we live.

Above and beyond the hardening of the bones, plus keeping them hard, is the need for lubrication for all the linings of the body. These facts are not even observed in the medical curriculum. It is time to include preventive medicine. Again I say, it is deplorable that the use of Cod Liver Oil has not been explored more fully.

With the unique method of taking the Cod

Liver Oil as I advocate, the unpleasant taste is gone. Therefore, the only undesirable part of Cod Liver Oil, the taste stigma, is now eradicated. I know Cod Liver Oil is on the rise.

You, the reader, may be due for a tasty surprise. There have been some newly created flavors of Cod Liver Oil: mint, wild cherry, strawberry and orange. You may even like it.

Here we've been discussing Cod Liver Oil as it <u>directly</u> relates to skin care. In the next chapter I am going to show you an indirect method of measuring both the quality and the effectiveness of your body lubricant supply.

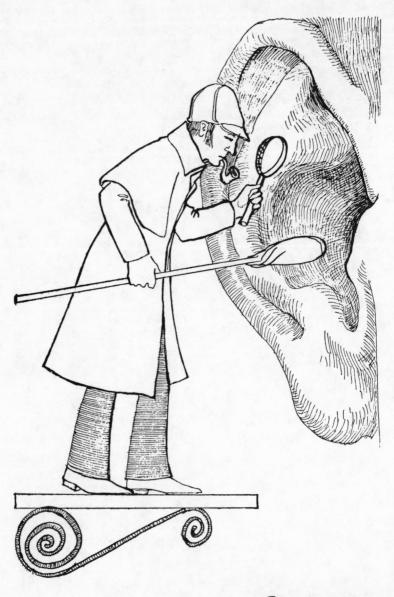

Earwax can tell us a great deal

13.

Earwax...the clue to lubrication and moisture in your skin

Sometimes, we must look to the lesser signs and signals our body gives us before we can accurately gauge its condition. For example, if we have bad breath, it can be indicative of poor digestion or other nominal problems. But, under certain circumstances, it <u>can</u> be one of the lesser symptoms of diabetes. Headaches, as another example, usually amount to nothing, but they <u>can</u> be a symptom of serious brain disorder.

Most often, bad breath and headache are simple problems which do not give us cause for alarm.

If they persist, of course, they should put us on guard.

Another of the body's telltale signals that should always put us on guard is an absence of or abnormality in our earwax. Earwax should be regarded as an essential substance. It can tell us a great deal about the function of our body.

The Basic Facts—Initial Earwax Research

Earwax is called cerumen, and, to this day, authorities disagree as to its precise function. During a Canadian lecture tour, I took out time to attend a seminar for Canada's otolaryngologists (ear and throat specialists). I asked one participant, "Doctor, is earwax good for you or bad for you?" He answered: "Earwax? I believe it is bad for you. If it gets impacted, it must be syringed out. I charge $25.00 to remove it."

Later, I confronted another doctor with the same question. He replied: "I believe earwax is good for you . . . because you are born with it, and it seems to protect you from fungus infections."

It later became obvious that most of the doctors had conflicting opinions. They had little knowledge about the manufacture, function, or purpose of earwax. It was all strange to them.

The microchemical analysis of earwax began to appear in scientific literature in the 1930s. The primary reason for research on earwax was to discover a cure for infections of the external ear.

In the *Index Medicus* there is a reference made to cerumen research done in Italy in 1962. At that time a causal relationship was found between cardiological disturbances and earwax.

Medical literature from Egypt was published in 1964. Dr. A. Yassia and others reported an association between otosclerosis (hardening of the bones in the ear) and cerumen. They found that in such a situation the earwax was sparse and usually very dry.

Drs. M. Miyahara and E. Matsunga were also studying earwax in Japan. Their report appeared in the "National Institute of Genetics" in 1966. They determined that wet cerumen was found more frequently in patients diagnosed with arteriosclerosis than in patients with other diseases.

In July of 1971, Dr. Nicholas P. Petrakis[*] wrote that earwax and genes had a common relationship. He found that wet (sticky) or dry (hard) cerumen is controlled by a pair of genes in which the allele for the wet type is dominant over that for the dry. In conducting research among Japanese women in San Francisco, he

[*] Dr. Petrakis is associated with the G. W. Hooper Foundation Department of International Health and Division of Ambulatory and Community Medicine at the University of California in San Francisco.

noted that those with wet cerumen presented roughly a twofold risk of developing cancer of the breast.

Dr. Henry P. Leis of New York Medical College, reporting to a 1974 convocation of the American College of Surgeons, told of a study made of breast cancer victims. He found that more than 70 percent of them had wet earwax. According to Dr. Leis, the same gene that regulates the structure and development of the breast is responsible for the type of earwax which a woman has. But Dr. Leis, like so many others, was failing to take nutrition into consideration during his research.

It is obvious that I am not alone when I emphasize the importance of earwax. Wet cerumen is involved in more than one disease, and it should always be taken as a warning sign. The condition of your skin is also a sign to be watched closely in such a case.

Make Your Own "Q-Tip"ᴿ Test

To understand better the significance of what you are about to read concerning cerumen, may I suggest that you examine your own ears. Do it now, first. This is one of your body's important oil lines and deserves constant checking.

Take a cotton-covered Q-tipᴿ, brush it into

and around your ear canals. When you remove it you will have conclusive proof of your personal oil supply. Here is what you are looking for:

The <u>color</u> of your earwax is a key factor. It should be golden yellow or light amber. This indicates your stomach is pumping oil to the proper places. Respect the color of your earwax on the Q-tip^R—it is important.

Next, check the <u>consistency</u> and <u>viscosity</u> of your earwax. It should be pasty, slightly tacky, and soft. Dry and cakey earwax is a sign of poor diet. Your body is telling you to select your dietary oils more carefully. Again, Cod Liver Oil can be greatly beneficial. But it must be used in the manner described in chapter twelve in order for it to be eventually converted into a proper form of earwax.

Continuing Ear Research

Dr. Albert P. Seltzer, writing in "American Practitioner's Transaction" in 1961, added a new dimension to the study of earwax. He wrote of the many doctors who came to him for personal consultation, complaining they had difficulty in hearing their own patients. They expressed the fear that they were losing their hearing.

Dr. Seltzer examined these doctor-patients

with an otoscope. He found accumulations of cerumen in their ears. Sometimes the accumulation
of waxy secretion had reached a point of impaction. Such a condition, of course, can cause limi-
tation of hearing, and even cause disturbing
noises. These "noises" are known as "tinnitus."

After careful removal of the earwax, the doctors tried to use their stethoscopes. Some of them
still experienced difficulty in hearing sub-aural
sounds.

Next, the stethoscope ear-pieces were examined. They were found to be filled with earwax.
When this secondary problem was relieved, full
hearing was restored.

Dr. Seltzer examined a total of sixty doctors.
Of these, 10 percent had impacted cerumen of
which they were entirely unaware.

Simultaneously, another doctor was hard at
work studying earwax problems. Dr. James Kawchak of the Ford Motor Company published his
findings in the *Journal of Occupational Medicine*.
His study was related to industrial health hazards.

It has been know for some time that the high
intensity of noise found in heavy industry can result in the loss of hearing, in fatigue, and in a general lessening of efficiency. At the same time it is
known that one of the means of maintaining peak
efficiency—whether in heavy industry or at desk

jobs—is to have full hearing. This called for the removal of excessive earwax.

Dr. Kawchak found ways to remove hardened earwax, but he ignored the dietary patterns which caused the impaction. He did report, however, that excessive earwax produced <u>subclinical conduction deafness.</u>

Dr. Kawchak's experimental research made no mention of the elements within the earwax.

Fortunately, at the same time, others were analyzing the chemistry of earwax. A leader in this field was Dr. F. B. De Jorge in the Department of Otorhinolaryngology at the University of San Paulo Medical School in Brazil.

He found that earwax contained many volatile substances, such as ash, sodium, potassium, calcium, magnesium, phosphorus, and copper.

He called attention to the high relative copper content in healthy cerumen. Copper is a trace mineral. It plays a role in many enzyme systems and is essential to the production of ribonucleic acid (RNA). Copper also aids in the development of bones, hair, nerves, and connective tissue. A deficiency of copper decreases absorption of iron and shortens the life span of red blood cells, thus causing anemia.

Furthermore, even though copper content in earwax is quite diffuse, it still plays a role in the aural conductivity which must precede good hearing.

Healthy earwax, then, is an indication that the body is receiving ample quantities of a very important basic element.

How Earwax Is Formed

Aural wax—cerumen—consists of a mixture of the secretions from the sebaceous and ceruminous glands of the external ear canal. Cerumen is a mixed product of these several glands.

If you haven't been cleaning your ears, at least occasionally, your earwax may appear to have too deep an amber color. This might be owing to oxidation of copper.

When you examine your own ears, the Q-tip^R may register streaky amounts. This is serious and indicates you are flirting with danger. I maintain nerve deafness is often caused by a lack of correct dietary oils. These are not reaching your ceruminous glands so as to form the sheath material which covers and protects the nerve tissues.

Dr. Samuel Kopetsky, an outstanding contributor to ear-related research, has written of the enzyme "cholinesterase" and its role in triggering sounds between the synapses of the human hearing system. The richest natural producers of cholinesterase are the B-complex vitamins, as found in Brewer's yeast. Brewer's yeast, then, can be helpful in the prevention of nerve deafness.

Nerve deafness, and even otosclerosis, can be prevented by proper diet. With the added use of Cod Liver Oil you should be able to acquire soft earwax within approximately six months.

Summary

Unfortunately, ear doctors seem not to understand the relationship between earwax and diet. For this reason, they usually cannot help one to achieve needed quantities of properly textured, properly colored cerumen.

Indeed, their primary concern seems to be removal of earwax. When the wax is cakey, or impacted, this is a good practice, but only then. Remember, also, that syringing out of earwax solves nothing basic.

To achieve soft, pasty, yellow, slightly tacky earwax, one must pay strict attention to diet. It takes a great deal of Cod Liver Oil to change the "ear-crankcase," and this must be taken but one tablespoon at a time (emulsified in milk, of course), over a period of from six to twelve months. At the same time, we should eat foods rich in copper: radishes, milk, organ meats, dry beans, salads. We should also eat foods rich in B-vitamins. Brewer's yeast is indicated.

Avoid ice creams, hydrogenated peanut butter, and margarines. Also avoid fried oils, which become metabolically inert oils in the body.

Do not be dismayed if earwax appears on your towel after a shower. This is normal. But do take the opportunity to check for consistency and color.

Do take special note (especially women) if earwax becomes liquid or runny. Remember the high incidence of breast cancer associated with such a condition discovered by researchers.

Next—the following chapter deals with the astounding power wielded over your skin—by the liquids you drink.

Following it to a T, can be the key, wait and see.

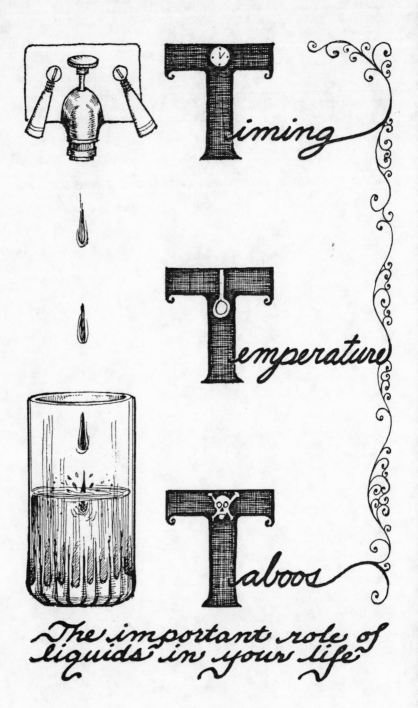

Timing

Temperature

Taboos

The important role of liquids in your life

14.

The three "T's"
Liquids... Timing,
Temperature,
and Taboos

Let's use some good old "horse sense." I believe in the old axiom that "You can lead a horse to water, but you can't make him drink."

By instinct, a horse knows enough not to drink polluted water. We should be so smart!

Do you realize that <u>most</u> man-made liquid concoctions are unfit to drink. They are usually polluted with chemicals, preservatives, and acids.

Too many people are completely unaware of the havoc that is wrought inside their own bodies when they indiscriminately drink the wrong liquids. In this chapter, I shall praise certain liquids, and damn most of the others, by name.

With continuing research—almost to the point of dedication—I have studied liquids of all types. I believe that I have arrived at some exciting conclusions. When I reveal them, here, the simplicity of my findings will make you wonder why man hasn't discovered these answers until now.

The Three T's Are Your Three Keys

To explain my theories about liquids—in simple, nonmedical terms—let me use my designation known as "THE THREE Ts."

They are: the Timing of when you drink liquids. . . the Temperature of those liquids when you drink them . . . and the Taboos of certain liquids taken with meals.

TIMING is critical to assimilation. In the process of digesting solids and liquids there is a sequence which must be followed.

Oil-bearing liquids—like milk and soup—are the ideal drinks to have with your meals. (As I pointed out in chapter eleven concerning cholesterol.) But the oil-free liquids—like water, coffee, and tea—should be consumed at least ten minutes before your meal. If not then, you can have the option to drink these liquids, providing you wait a minimum of three hours after your meal.

You should always remember one basic fact: The liquids that you drink with your meals control the delivery of oil into your blood stream.

Whether or not you will have good lubrication and moisturization of your skin depends on you. There must be an orderly sequence for your "intake" of oil-bearing liquids.

This may sound like too simple an act to produce such positive results. But this dietary recommendation really works. Why? Because your skin has been begging for its vital oil nutrients. Too often, the oils were routed into the liver, because the proper sequence of timing was ignored.

TEMPERATURE of liquids—while you are consuming them—can vitally affect your health. Guidance from doctors on the subject of temperature of liquids has been sadly lacking. So, let me explain a few simple truths. . . .

Most of us know that our body temperature is around 98.6. When you consume iced liquids, within moments the body temperature drops. The heart responds by pumping faster, and the whole body is jolted.

Any iced drink, taken on an empty stomach, is punishing enough. But it is even worse when food is already in your stomach. The iced bever-

age causes the oils in your stomach to become solidified. This is the reverse of good digestion. You
are causing a traumatic burden on your gall bladder and your pancreas.

Therefore, you can now see that there is a
direct relationship between the drinking of iced
liquids and the condition of your skin.

Why let iced beverages cause the essential
fatty acids needed by your skin to be routed into
the liver?

If these fatty acids do go into your liver, they
may be more than what your liver can handle. In
that event they will merely show up in your waistline . . . make you fat.

At the same time, your skin will be deprived
of many oils (containing precious Vitamin A)
and you will not be able to achieve supple skin.

TABOOS are necessary in regard to drinking
liquids. The following paragraphs will list the
various liquids which you should avoid.

Let's start with the most injurious ones.

Carbonated Soft Drinks. The harmful substances in these drinks play a devastating role in
skin diseases. They help to cause acne, eczema,
dermatitis, psoriasis, skin cancer, and many other
afflictions.

I believe—as many nutrition experts do—
that most carbonated drinks contain damaging
synthetic chemical acids and gaseous elements. I
am particularly concerned about the phosphoric

acid, the tartaric acid, and the synthetic citric acid found in most soft drinks. These acids are vicious enemies of healthy skin.

Tannic Acid Tea. While making leather goods, the tanning industry uses tannic to "dry out" the oils in the skin of animals. Long-term tea drinkers, from my observations, have the dryest and most wrinkled skin of any human beings anywhere. Adding sugar and lemon to tea, as is usually done, only compounds the problem.

There is now available, in health food stores, a variety of herb teas. These are beneficial.

Even with herb tea, drink it only when your stomach is empty, and not with meals.

Acetic Acid Vinegars. The vinegar you consume—in the form of dressing with salads—is acceptable in my dietary program. Because you are chewing your salad and, therefore, the acetic acid in the vinegar is neutralized by the saliva. Vinegar, brought into your body this way, can be an ally. It is when you drink vinegar that it becomes damaging.

Some books on health actually recommend that the reader should drink vinegar—or even vinegar and honey. I maintain that the long-term consumption of vinegar in this manner will result in too high an acid level in your blood stream. The unfortunate result will be more dryness in your skin.

Powdered "Imitation" Drinks. Mixes of synthetic powders (as an aide to keep cool) have zero value from a nutritional point of view. These drinks provide your body with no real nourishment. As a matter of fact, these unnatural, man-made products are difficult for the body to assimilate and use. For a lustrous skin, stay away from these powdered concoctions.

Frozen Fruit Juices. These refrigerated liquids are quite damaging, in my opinion, because they lack enzymes. And, remember, an abundant supply of enzymes is one way to prevent dry and wrinkled skin.

Frozen fruit juices also create a higher level of acids than is desirable. If you like the taste of oranges, grapefruit, apples, etc., then eat the entire fruit rather than drinking them in juice form.

Nonfat Milk. This is an altered food, and it does little for your skin. With the fat having been drained out, this type of milk can hardly be expected to add the right lubricating oils to your system. Whole milk is a far better choice, if you drink it according to the menu plan set up in chapter fifteen.

Fresh Prepared Juices. Fruit and vegetable juices—even if they are prepared fresh—are not too beneficial. As I recommended before, eat the entire fruit or vegetable, instead of drinking just the juices. When we eat fruits or vegetables in their whole state, the neutralizing salts in our

saliva will prepare these foods for easy digestibil-
ity. If you just gulp down the juices, these liquids
miss the good work which can be done by your
saliva. Without help from your saliva, these
quickly-consumed juices have not been neutralized and therefore present a problem for your
skin.

How About "The Happy Hour" Drinks?

When it's "Cocktail Time" you do not have
to become a party pooper. Surprise! I am not going to add all alcoholic beverages to my list of
taboo liquids.

Alcohol, wine, and beer are permitted. As
long as you drink with moderation, and according
to a few simple dietary rules. Obviously, you
should not go out and drink it up until you get a
skin-full.

In addition to being cautious about the
amount of liquor which you drink, watch the way
that you consume such liquids.

Again—even with alcohol, wine, and beer—
you should pay attention to timing and temperature. For all three of these types of beverages, the
following instructions apply:

Cocktails—mixed drinks, containing ice
cubes—are wrong if you have food in your stomach. If you must drink alcohol, drink it straight.

Skip the ice cubes. No club soda, tonic water, or other mixes, and try to limit yourself to one shot per day. Again, ice is only permissible if your stomach is empty.

Wine consumption should be limited to about four ounces per day. Please drink it at room temperature, and only before meals. Do not drink wine with, or after the meal.

Beer is naturally carbonated, so at least it doesn't contain the chemical acids or synthetic acids found in some soft drinks. An eleven-ounce bottle of beer once in a while is not going to damage, drastically, your chances for a healthy skin. We recommend the bottled beer because preservatives are added to the cans.

Note: For all of the above beverages, the same timing is important. It's as simple as a-b-c to remember. Never drink any of these liquids with meals. Enjoy them, but only at LEAST TEN MINUTES BEFORE A MEAL . . . OR, THREE HOURS AFTER A MEAL.

If you agree with the concepts which I have outlined in this chapter, these alcoholic beverages will be the least harmful to your body.

By themselves, these rules are critical. But to gain the maximum potential they have to be incorporated in a total nutrition program.

The following chapter does this for you.

Part Four

HOW TO AVOID MALNOURISHMENT OF YOUR SKIN

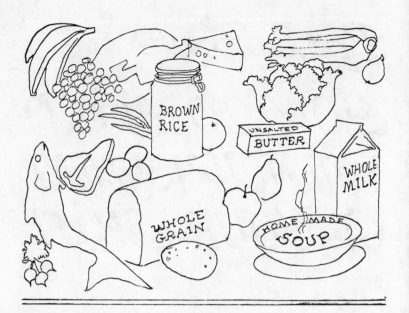

Which is your diet?

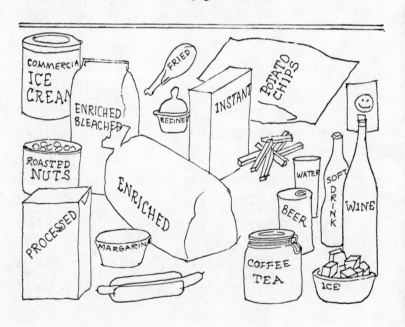

15.

Prime Nutrition Menus & Recipes

for normal, dry and dry-oily (combination) skin

I am often asked, "What is a balanced diet?" Obviously, a properly balanced diet is one that contains everything the body needs; proteins, fats, carbohydrates, minerals, vitamins. These must be in proper proportion, and should come, so far as is possible, from natural sources.

However, the human body is a remarkably adaptive instrument and it can make certain adjustments to correct periodic dietary mismanagement. It has the capacity to compensate for excesses so that they have no immediate bad effect. It also has the capacity to tide us over whenever there is a temporary lacking of necessary nutrients in our diet.

Often as not, we do receive many of the foods we need in our daily diets, although we have made no conscious effort to do so. But it is not only a matter of using proper base foods. The whole secret lies in the manner in which these foods are assimilated. And assimilation is almost completely controlled by the liquids we drink, and when we drink them. As I have said before, this is the key, the whole and single key, to good nutrition. It is the key which is missing from all other manuals on nutrition.

The greatly commercial enterprise of feeding billions—while at the same time making a tidy profit—has given rise to a vast "processed food" industry. As a result, Americans—and other modern societies—have developed some highly dangerous eating habits, most of which center about these processed foods.

Any chemical adulteration of foods unbalances nature. Any unnatural chemical addition to our food becomes an unnatural addition to our diet, because we eat it.

Certain foods are rendered virtually useless in the course of "processing" for the mass market. Take cereals, for instance. They are exploded from cannons, puffed with air, saturated with preservatives, dunked and lathered with sugar, and then packaged in such a way that children—whose bodies most need good nourishment—cannot resist them. And the process must be profitable. An entire television industry-within-an-industry has been created to sell these cereals.

Two Nutritional Stop-Signs

Two words, more than any other, should serve as nutritional stop-signs in our diets. One is "refined," the other is "enriched." Refined sugars and flours have been stripped of nutrients so as to reduce the product to a simple, easy-to-store-and-ship base carbohydrate. "Enriched" bread is really a mockery upon the language. First, processed flours are used, from which have already been extracted about 98 percent of the basic natural nutrients, and to which, just before marketing, about 2 percent of these nutrients have been restored. The buyer ends up with a product which has about 4 percent of its original nutrients, and which, on this account, is labeled "enriched." To add insult to injury, we are charged extra for this!

Allergies

One of the by-products of our high-speed dietary blunders is allergy. Processed foods—unnatural foods—have a tendency to weaken body tolerances to all allergens. Food allergies themselves, which seem to be on the rise, are thought by many experts to be triggered by chemical adulteration.

There is no reason for any thinking person to be taken in by the TV brain-washing sponsored by dollar-hungry food-processing corporations. It is to these corporations' benefit to find ways to package foods so they will not deteriorate on the shelf. But that doesn't mean you have to buy them.

Remember the nutritional taboos. Beware of processed foods. Understand the true meaning of "enriched" and "refined." White sugar, white flour, and their resulting products (white bread, especially) are nonnutritious, useless, and often injurious to the human body.

The Balanced Diet

The truly balanced diet need not be the same for everyone. A balance can be maintained and one's personal tastes satisfied. You can be a vegetarian, a carnivore, you can be a lover of fish or nuts or berries, and still achieve a harmonious balance.

I have compiled here three groups of menus. The first is a group of day-by-day menus for normal skin, the second is for dry skin, and the third for oily-dry (combination) skin.

Remember always that a diet is only what you make of it. The discipline that goes into the diet, and the length of time it is used, are usually the factors which determine its efficacy.

The following menus include information on salad-making, salad dressings, soups, and wholesome desserts.

If you have weight problems—over or under —the same foodstuffs are suggested, with the size of the portions adjusted to fit your needs.

These menus can be the key to good health and a supple, lustrous skin—all without sacrifice of enjoyment.

Above all, remember, these menus are not meant to be inflexible. Make sensible substitutions so as to please your own tastes.

So . . . read on. Carve out for yourself a bountiful table of good food. The way to a lovely skin is through your stomach.

Happy eating!

A WEEK'S GUIDE OF DAILY MENUS FOR NORMAL SKIN

MONDAY

Upon arising: One or two glasses of water (tap or bottle).
Twenty minutes later: Cod Liver Oil MINI-MILKSHAKE* (see chapter six).
One hour later:

BREAKFAST

Orange	1, sliced
Eggs	1 or 2, softboiled or poached
Whole Wheat English Muffin	1, toasted
Butter	1 pat
Whole Milk	8 ounces

LUNCH

Salad (Lettuce, tomato, celery, and cucumber)	generous serving (sprinkle with sunflower, sesame, or pumpkin seeds)
Cottage Cheese	1 scoop, mixed with one tbsp. yogurt
Whole Wheat Bread	1 or 2 slices
Butter	1 pat
Whole Milk	8 ounces

DINNER

Upside-Down Vegetable Salad	generous serving (see this chapter)
Calves Liver	4 to 6 ounces, broiled
Onions	½ cup, sauteed
String Beans	½ cup, steamed
Baked Potato	1, medium
Butter	1 pat
Whole Milk	8 ounces
Melon, in season, or fresh fruit	

* For those who prefer taking Cod Liver Oil the night before rather than the morning, this is permissible, provided it is taken 4 or more hours after last solid-food intake.

TUESDAY

Upon arising: One or two glasses of water (tap or bottle).
Twenty minutes later: Cod Liver Oil MINI-MILKSHAKE.*
One hour later:

BREAKFAST

Black Mission Figs	3
Oatmeal, cooked	1 cup
Wheat Germ, raw	1 tbsp., sprinkled on oatmeal
Butter	1 pat
Whole Milk	8 ounces

LUNCH

Homemade Vegetable Soup	1 bowl
Hamburger	one 3- to 4-ounce patty
Whole Wheat Hamburger Bun	1, lined with alfalfa sprouts
Onion	1 slice, on hamburger
Whole Milk	8 ounces

DINNER

Upside-Down Vegetable Salad	generous serving
Roast Beef	4 to 6 ounces, rare
Broccoli	½ cup, steamed
Brown Rice	½ cup
Whole Milk	8 ounces
Fresh Fruit	
* See "Monday."	

WEDNESDAY

Upon arising: One or two glasses of water (tap or bottle).
Twenty minutes later: Cod liver Oil MINI-MILKSHAKE.*
One hour later:

BREAKFAST

Prunes	3 or 4
Dry Wheat Flakes	1 bowl
Wheat Germ, raw	1 tbsp., on flakes
Banana, sliced	1
Whole Milk	8 ounces

LUNCH

Onion Soup	1 cup
Whole Wheat Crackers	4
Fresh Fruit Salad	1 apple, ½ cup blueberries, 2 figs, or 1 small banana
Black Raisins	¼ cup
Yogurt, for dressing	½ cup
Sunflower and Pumpkin Seeds	sprinkle over salad
Whole Milk	8 ounces

DINNER

Upside-Down Vegetable Salad	generous serving
Lamb Chops	1 large or 2 small, broiled
Zucchini Squash	1 cup, steamed
Baked Potato	1, medium
Butter	1 pat
Whole Milk	8 ounces
Fresh Fruit	
* See "Monday."	

THURSDAY

Upon arising: One or two glasses of water (tap or bottle).
Twenty minutes later: Cod Liver Oil MINI-MILKSHAKE.*
One hour later:

BREAKFAST

Orange	1, sliced
Egg—omelet	1 or 2
Whole Wheat Bread	1 or 2 slices
Butter	1 pat
Whole Milk	8 ounces

LUNCH

Salad (lettuce, radishes, celery, alfalfa sprouts, tomato)	small
Roast Beef Sandwich	4 ounces, rare, on whole wheat bread
Butter	1 pat, or substitute mayonnaise
Whole Milk	8 ounces

DINNER

Upside-Down Salad	generous serving
Trout	6 ounces, broiled
Onions and Tomatoes	fresh, 4 ounces, sauteed
String Beans	½ cup, steamed
Brown Rice	½ cup
Butter	1 pat
Whole Milk	8 ounces
Fresh Fruit	

* See "Monday."

FRIDAY

Upon arising: One or two glasses of water (tap or bottle).
Twenty minutes later: Cod Liver Oil MINI-MILKSHAKE.*
One hour later:

BREAKFAST

Pink Grapefruit	½
Whole Wheat Dry Cereal	Medium bowl (or rice, oat, or rye flks)
Raw Wheat Germ	1 tbsp.
Banana	1, small, sliced
Whole Milk	8 ounces

LUNCH

Fish and Vegetable Chowder	1 bowl
Egg Salad Sandwich	whole wheat bread, with alfalfa sprouts and sliced tomatoes
Whole Milk	8 ounces

DINNER

Upside-Down Salad	generous serving
Salmon	4 to 6 ounces, poached or broiled
Squash, young	½ cup, steamed
Baked Potato	1, medium
Butter	1 pat
Whole Milk	8 ounces
Fresh Fruit	

    * See "Monday."

SATURDAY

Upon arising: One or two glasses of water (tap or bottle).
Twenty minutes later: Cod Liver Oil MINI-MILKSHAKE.*
One hour later:

BREAKFAST

Black Mission Figs	3
Soya and Wheat Cereal	cooked, 1 cup
Raw Wheat Germ	1 tbsp.
Butter	1 pat
Whole Milk	8 ounces

LUNCH

Lentil Soup	1 bowl
Salad	small; lettuce, green onions, tomato, celery, raw white turnip
Chicken Liver and Egg Omelet	4 ounces
Whole Wheat Bread	1 slice
Whole Milk	8 ounces

DINNER

Upside-Down Salad	generous serving
Steak	4 to 6 ounces, lean, broiled
Cauliflower	½ cup
Acorn Squash	½, baked
Butter	1 pat
Whole Milk	8 ounces
Fresh Fruit	

    * See "Monday."

SUNDAY

Upon arising: One or two glasses of water (tap or bottle).
Twenty minutes later: Cod Liver Oil MINI-MILKSHAKE.*
One hour later:

BREAKFAST

Orange	1, sliced
Canadian Bacon or Lean Ham	3 ounces
Eggs	2, poached
Whole Wheat Bread	1 or 2 slices
Butter	1 pat
Whole Milk	8 ounces

LUNCH

Upside-Down Salad	generous serving
Cottage Cheese	1 cup
Apple	1
Whole Milk	8 ounces

DINNER

Soup	1 cup
Roast Chicken	
Cranberry Sauce	
Sweet Potato	one, medium
Brussel Sprouts	½ cup
Celery	
Whole Milk	8 ounces

    * See "Monday."

The Dry-skin Diet

Before proceeding to the menus for a dry skin, let me make some general comments about dieting.

Most diets, and especially those appearing here, are not governed by a time limit. They can easily become lifetime regimens. As a rule, the reason for dieting in the first place will determine the optimum length of time one should remain on it. Here I am addressing myself to skin care, and it is a simple matter to check for improvements. You will have no difficulty knowing when your dry skin has regained its natural pliancy. But that state of improvement should not be interpreted as meaning you may now go berserk with foodless food. What you have been doing was correct. You now know a way of life which leads to a soft, supple, healthy-appearing skin.

The Dry-Skin Diet differs from others in that Vitamin A capsules (up to 10,000 units) are added at each breakfast. The foods themselves are also of high Vitamin A content. The capsules should be taken with the milk at the close of the meal—never with water.

A WEEK'S GUIDE OF DAILY MENUS FOR OVERCOMING DRY SKIN

MONDAY

Upon arising: One or two glasses of water (tap or bottle).
Twenty minutes later: Cod Liver Oil MINI-MILKSHAKE* (see chapter six).
One hour later:

BREAKFAST

Prunes	4 or 5
Eggs	1 or 2, soft boiled
Whole Wheat Bread	1 or 2 slices
Butter	1 pat
Whole Milk	8 ounces
Vitamin A Capsule	up to 10,000 units

LUNCH

Beef Vegetable Soup	1 cup
Cheddar Cheese Sandwich	whole wheat bread
Alfalfa Sprouts	
Sliced Tomatoes	
Carrot Spears	
Celery Sticks	
Whole Milk	8 ounces

DINNER

Upside-Down Salad	generous serving
Halibut	4 to 6 ounces, broiled
Onions and Tomatoes	½ cup, sauteed
Pumpkin Squash	½ cup, steamed
Butter	1 pat
Whole Milk	8 ounces
Melon in season, or other fresh fruit	

* For those who prefer taking Cod Liver Oil the night before, rather than in the morning, this is permissible, provided it is taken 4 or more hours after last solid-food intake.

TUESDAY

Upon arising: One or two glasses of water (tap or bottle).
Twenty minutes later: Cod Liver Oil MINI-MILKSHAKE*
One hour later:

BREAKFAST

Whole Wheat Dry Cereal	1 bowl
Raw Wheat Germ	2 tbsp.
Banana	1, sliced
Apricots	2, fresh or dried
Whole Milk	8 ounces
Vitamin A	up to 10,000 units

LUNCH

Salad (escarole, cherry tomatoes, bean sprouts, carrot spears)	
Yogurt, for dressing	¼ cup
Egg—omelet	1 or 2, with Swiss cheese
Whole Wheat Bread	1 or 2 slices
Butter	1 pat
Whole Milk	8 ounces

DINNER

Upside-Down Salad	generous serving
Beef Kidney	4 to 6 ounces, braised
Kale	½ cup, steamed
Onions and Green Pepper	½ cup, sauteed
Brown Rice	½ cup, steamed
Butter	1 pat
Whole Milk	8 ounces
Fresh pineapple slices	

* See "Monday."

WEDNESDAY

Upon arising: One or two glasses of water (tap or bottle).
Twenty minutes later: Cod Liver Oil MINI-MILKSHAKE*
One hour later:

BREAKFAST

Orange or Tangerine	1
Cornmeal Mush Cereal	6 ounces
Sesame Seeds	1 tbsp., sprinkled on cereal
Butter	1 pat
Whole Milk	8 ounces
Vitamin A	up to 10,000 units

LUNCH

Oyster Stew (with milk)	one eight-ounce bowl
Vegetable Salad (green lettuce, celery, carrot sticks, tomato, avocado wedge)	
Cottage Cheese	1 scoop
Pumpkin Seeds	sprinkle on salad
Whole Milk	4 ounces

DINNER

Roast Beef	4 to 6 ounces, rare
Kale	½ cup, steamed
Corn	½ cup, steamed
Potato	1, baked
Butter	1 pat
Whole Milk	8 ounces
Fresh Fruit	
* See "Monday."	

THURSDAY

Upon arising: One or two glasses of water (tap or bottle).
Twenty minutes later: Cod Liver Oil MINI-MILKSHAKE*
One hour later:

BREAKFAST

Papaya	½
Millet Flakes	1 bowl
Raisins	2 tbsp.
Whole Milk	8 ounces
Vitamin A	up to 10,000 units

LUNCH

Fruit Salad	3 fresh or dried apricots, diced apple, sliced banana, persimmons
Yogurt	¼ cup, on salad
Sunflower and Sesame Seeds	sprinkle on salad
Whole Milk	6 ounces

DINNER

Upside-Down Salad	generous serving
Calves Liver	4 to 6 ounces, broiled
Onions	4 ounces, sautéed
Swiss Chard	½ cup, steamed
Sweet Potato	1, baked
Whole Milk	8 ounces
Homemade Custard	small portion
* See "Monday."	

FRIDAY

Upon arising: One or two glasses of water (tap or bottle).
Twenty minutes later: Cod Liver Oil MINI-MILKSHAKE*
One hour later:

BREAKFAST

Black Mission Figs	3 or 4
Poached Eggs	1 or 2
Whole Wheat English Muffin	1
Butter	1 pat
Milk	8 ounces
Vitamin A	up to 10,000 units

LUNCH

Clam Chowder	8-ounce bowl
Swiss Cheese Sandwich	whole wheat bread, alfalfa sprouts, sliced tomatoes, fresh parsley
Whole Milk	6 ounces

DINNER

Upside-Down Salad	generous serving
Salmon	4 to 6 ounces, broiled
Yellow Summer Squash	¼ cup
Zucchini Squash	¼ cup
Brown Rice	1 cup
Whole Milk	8 ounces
Fresh Fruit	
* See "Monday."	

SATURDAY

Upon arising: One or two glasses of water (tap or bottle).
Twenty minutes later: Cod Liver Oil MINI-MILKSHAKE*
One hour later:

BREAKFAST

Pink Grapefruit	½
Oatmeal or Rye Cereal	1 bowl, cooked
Sesame Seeds	2 tbsp., sprinkle on cereal
Butter	1 pat
Whole Milk	8 ounces
Vitamin A	up to 10,000 units

LUNCH

Salad (green lettuce, raw spinach, tomatoes, green onions, diced white turnip)	
Hamburger Patty	3 or 4 ounce
Whole Wheat Hamburger Bun	lined with alfalfa sprouts
Whole Milk	8 ounces

DINNER

Upside-Down Salad	generous serving
Roast Leg of Lamb	4 to 6 ounces
Sweet Potato	1, baked
String Beans	½ cup, steamed
Butter	1 pat
Whole Milk	8 ounces
Fresh Fruit	
* See "Monday."	

SUNDAY

Upon arising: One or two glasses of water (tap or bottle).
Twenty minutes later: Cod Liver Oil MINI-MILKSHAKE*
One hour later:

BREAKFAST

Orange or Tangerine	1
Egg—omelet	1 or 2, with chicken livers
Whole Wheat Bread	1 or 2 slices
Butter	1 pat
Whole Milk	8 ounces
Vitamin A	up to 10,000 units

LUNCH

Fruit Salad (sliced banana, grapes, melon, cherries, apricots or any fruit in season)	
Yogurt	¼ cup
Mixed Almond Meal	
Cottage Cheese	¼ cup
Whole Wheat Crackers	4 to 6
Whole Milk	6 ounces

DINNER

Upside-Down Salad	generous serving
Onion Soup	6-ounce cup
Chicken or Other Fowl	4 to 6 ounces, roasted or broiled
Vegtables (brussel sprouts, onions, or mushrooms, steamed)	1 cup
Brown Rice	½ cup
Whole Milk	8 ounces
Tapioca Egg Pudding	

* See "Monday."

ADDITIONAL OPTIONAL FOODS RICH IN VITAMIN A

VEGETABLES

Pumpkin	Raw Green Onions
Escarole	Parsley
Kale	Fresh Peas, steamed
Okra, steamed	Carrots, raw or steamed
Sweet Potatoes	Peppers
Spinach	Green Beans
Winter Squash	Asparagus
Summer Squash	Uncooked Bean Sprouts
Tomatoes	Beet Greens, steamed
Turnip Greens, steamed	Broccoli, steamed
Watercress	Brussel Sprouts, steamed
Avocado	Swiss Chard, steamed
Dandelion Greens, steamed	Collards, steamed
Green Leaf Lettuce	Corn, steamed
Mustard Greens, steamed	

FRUITS

Cherries
Peaches
Apricots
Persimmons
Papaya
Pears
Pineapple

Prunes
Raspberries
Tangerines
Watermelon
Fresh Oranges
Cantaloupe

MEATS

Kidneys, braised
Beef Liver
Calves' Liver
Liverwurst
Chicken Livers
Fowl

FISH

Halibut
Swordfish
Codfish
Raw Oysters
Eels
Crabs

SOUPS

Beef Vegetable
Clam Chowder
Oyster Stew with Milk
Vegetable

DESSERTS

Custard
Ice Cream
Tapioca Pudding
Rice Pudding

DAIRY FOODS

Cow's Whole Milk
Goat's Milk
Heavy Sweet Cream
Yogurt
Cottage Cheese
Butter
Aged Cheeses (not lofat)

GRAINS

Rice

Dry-oily (Combination) Skin

No other book has ever addressed itself solely
to a dietary regimen aimed at correcting "dry" or
"oily-dry" skin. People mistakenly believe that
"oily" skin can be corrected simply by extracting
oils from their diets. Well, it just doesn't work that
way. The skin is always in great need of oils, but
since it is a greatly selective organ, it will reject
inferior, cooked, or vitaminless oils. (Vitamin
"A"—the "oiler"—and essential fatty acids—"the
healer"—must both be present.)

To combat <u>Dry-Oily</u> skin, we need foods rich in the B-complex vitamins. Especially, we require a daily supplement of B₆ (pyridoxine) which will help achieve the <u>Double Bond Exchange</u> (discussed earlier in chapter seven, "What if You Have Both Dry and Oily Skin?").

I have also added a list of various foods rich in B vitamins to be used as alternatives in the daily diets.

The Dry-Oily (Combination) Skin Diet is altogether different from those preceding. The foods in the following menus are rich in Vitamin B. Each breakfast calls for supplementary Vitamin B Complex, which contains the B₆ (pyridoxine) mentioned above. These, too, must be taken with milk at the close of the meal, not with water.

A WEEK'S GUIDE OF DAILY MENUS FOR DRY-OILY (COMBINATION) SKIN

MONDAY

Upon arising: One or two glasses of water (tap or bottle).
Twenty minutes later: Cod Liver Oil MINI-MILKSHAKE* (see chapter six).
One hour later:

BREAKFAST

Black Mission Figs	4
Soya, Wheat Cereal	1 bowl, cooked
Wheat Germ	1 tbsp., sprinkled on cereal
Butter	1 pat
Whole Milk	8 ounces
Vitamin B-Complex	25 to 50 milligrams

LUNCH

Homemade Lentil Soup	4-ounce bowl
Lean Hamburger	3- or 4-ounce patty, mixed with one tsp. rice polishings and one tsp. sunflower seed meal, broiled rare
Whole Wheat Hamburger Bun	lined with slice of raw onion and alfalfa sprouts
Whole Milk	8 ounces

DINNER

Upside-Down Salad	generous serving
Heart	4 to 6 ounces, braised
Onions, Green Peppers, and Tomatoes	4 to 8 ounces, sauteed
Broccoli	½ cup, steamed
Sweet Yam	1, baked
Whole Milk	8 ounces
Fresh Fruit in Season	

* For those who prefer taking Cod Liver Oil the night before, rather than in the morning, this is permissible, provided it is taken 4 or more hours after last solid-food intake.

TUESDAY

Upon arising: One or two glasses of water (tap or bottle).
Twenty minutes later: Cod Liver Oil MINI-MILKSHAKE.*
One hour later:

BREAKFAST

Pink Grapefruit	½
Eggs	1 or 2, soft boiled
Pumpkin Seed Meal	1 tsp., atop eggs
Whole Wheat Bread	1 or 2 slices
Butter	1 pat
Whole Milk	8 ounces
Vitamin B-Complex	25 to 50 milligrams

LUNCH

Vegetable Barley Soup	1 small cup
Salad (green lettuce, celery, cucumbers, radishes, tomatoes, green onions)	
Cottage Cheese	1 scoop
Pumpkin, Sunflower, and Wheat Germ	sprinkled over salad
Whole Wheat Crackers	2 to 4
Whole Milk	6 ounces

DINNER

Upside-Down Salad	generous serving
Baby Beef or Calves' Liver	4 to 6 ounces, broiled
Onions and Mushrooms	4 to 6 ounces, sautéed
Fresh Lima Beans	½ cup, steamed
Brown Rice	½ cup
Whole Milk	8 ounces
Fresh Fruit in Season	

* See "Monday."

WEDNESDAY

Upon arising: One or two glasses of water (tap or bottle).
Twenty minutes later: Cod Liver Oil MINI-MILKSHAKE.*
One hour later:

BREAKFAST

Prunes	4 or 5
Whole Wheat Dry Cereal	1 bowl
Wheat Germ	1 tbsp., atop cereal
Rice Polishings	1 tsp., atop cereal
Banana	1, sliced
Whole milk	8 ounces
Vitamin B-Complex	25 to 50 milligrams

LUNCH

Fresh Fruit Salad (diced apple, pear, papaya, melon, apricots, or fruits in season)	
Yogurt	½ cup, mixed with sunflower, sesame, and pumpkin seeds
Whole Milk	6 ounces

DINNER

Upside-Down Salad	generous serving
Flounder	4 to 6 ounces, broiled
Onions, green peppers and tomatoes	½ cup, sautéed
String Beans	½ cup, steamed
Potato	1, baked
Butter	1 pat
Whole Milk	8 ounces
Fresh Fruit	

* See "Monday."

THURSDAY

Upon arising: One or two glasses of water (tap or bottle).
Twenty minutes later: Cod Liver Oil MINI-MILKSHAKE.*
One hour later:

BREAKFAST

Orange	1, sliced
Oatmeal	1 bowl, cooked
Wheat Germ	1 tbsp., atop cereal
Rice Polishings	1 tsp., atop cereal
Whole Milk	8 ounces
Vitamin B-Complex	25 to 50 milligrams

LUNCH

Beef-Vegetable Soup	1 cup
Eggs—omelet	1 or 2, with cheddar cheese
Whole Wheat Bread	1 or 2 slices
Whole Milk	6 ounces

DINNER

Upside-Down Salad	generous serving
Roast Beef	4 to 6 ounces, rare
Zucchini Squash and Young Summer Squash	4 to 6 ounces, steamed
Potato	1, baked
Whole Milk	8 ounces
Fresh Fruit	

    * See "Monday."

FRIDAY

Upon arising: One or two glasses of water (tap or bottle).
Twenty minutes later: Cod Liver Oil MINI-MILKSHAKE.*
One hour later:

BREAKFAST

Black Mission Figs	4
Corn Meal Mush Cereal	1 bowl
Wheat Germ	1 tbsp., atop cereal
Whole Milk	8 ounces
Vitamin B-Complex	25 to 50 milligrams

LUNCH

Fish-Vegetable Chowder	1 cup
Swiss Cheese Sandwich	whole wheat bread, alfalfa sprouts, one tbsp. pumpkin seed meal, sliced tomato, slice raw onion
Whole Milk	8 ounces

DINNER

Upside-Down Salad	generous serving
Salmon	4 to 6 ounces, broiled
Cauliflower	½ cup, steamed
Sweet Potato	one, baked
Whole Milk	8 ounces
Fresh Fruit	

    * See "Monday."

SATURDAY

Upon arising: One or two glasses of water (tap or bottle).
Twenty minutes later: Cod Liver Oil MINI-MILKSHAKE.*
One hour later:

BREAKFAST

Dried Apricots	4 to 6, soaked overnight
Cooked Rye Cereal	1 bowl
Wheat Germ	1 tbsp., atop cereal
Rice Polishings	1 tsp., atop cereal
Whole Milk	8 ounces
Vitamin B-Complex	25 to 50 milligrams

LUNCH

Onion Soup	1 cup
Eggs—omelet	1 or 2, with 2 or 3 ounces chicken livers
Whole Wheat Bread	1 slice
Butter	1 pat
Whole Milk	8 ounces

DINNER

Upside-Down Salad	generous serving
Roast Leg of Lamb	4 to 6 ounces
Onions, Green Peppers, and Mushrooms	½ cup, sautéed
Swiss Chard	½ cup, steamed
Fresh Corn	½ cup, cut off kernel, steamed; or on the cob, steamed
Whole Milk	8 ounces
Fresh Fruit	
* See "Monday."	

SUNDAY

Upon arising: One or two glasses of water (tap or bottle).
Twenty minutes later: Cod Liver Oil MINI-MILKSHAKE.*
One hour later:

BREAKFAST

Fresh Strawberries or Fresh Blueberries	1 bowl, in season
Fresh Sweet Cream or Milk	enough to pour over fruit
Soya Bread French Toast	1 or 2 slices
Whole Milk	6 ounces
Vitamin B-Complex	25 to 50 milligrams

LUNCH

Fresh Fruit Salad (melon, grapes, persimmon, and banana, in season)	
Yogurt	½ cup, mixed with one tsp. each almond meal and sunflower seed meal, atop salad
Whole Wheat Crackers	2 to 4
Whole Milk	6 ounces

DINNER

Upside-Down Salad	generous serving
Roast Chicken, Duck, or Turkey	4 to 6 ounces
Onions and Mushrooms	½ cup, sauteed
Brussel Sprouts	½ cup, steamed
Brown or Wild Rice	½ cup
Whole Milk	8 ounces
Tapioca Pudding	1 dessert cup
* See "Monday."	

ADDITIONAL OPTIONAL FOODS RICH IN VITAMIN B

VEGETABLES

Tomatoes
Peas
Turnip Greens
Mustard Greens
Swiss Chard
Celery
Potatoes
Carrots
Cabbage
Beets
Beet Leaves
Cauliflower
Lettuce, green leaf
Broccoli

Onions
Peppers
Corn
String Beans
Mushrooms
Sweet Potatoes
Zucchini
Kale
Asparagus
Endive
Spinach
Radishes
Parsley

FRUITS

Grapefruit
Lemons
Oranges
Bananas
Pineapple
Apples
Melon
Peaches

Avocados
Grapes
Prunes
Dates
Cherries
Pears
Strawberries
Cantaloupe

MEAT AND POULTRY

Beef
Liver (Beef and Calf)
Kidney
Heart
Beef Tongue
Muscle Meats
Brains
Chicken
Chicken Livers
Turkey
Lamb
Veal

FISH AND SEAFOOD

Swordfish
Tuna
Shad
Salmon
Mackerel
Halibut
Oysters

MISCELLANEOUS

Pecans
Sunflower Seeds
Sesame Seeds
Peanuts
Cashews
Almonds
Yeast
Lentils
Molasses
Eggs
Soy Beans
Walnuts
Cow's Milk
Goat's Milk
Cheese

CEREALS AND GRAINS

Bran
Whole Wheat Bread
Wheat Germ
Brown Rice
Rice Polish
Rice Bran

RECIPES

FOR SALAD, SALAD DRESSINGS, SAUCES, SOUPS, AND DESSERTS

Following are some unique and nutritionally beneficial recipes not to be found in any of the conventional cookbooks.

I have assembled these recipes with an eye toward both simplicity and taste appeal. They are primarily aimed at high nutritive value, which is achieved through minimum cooking.

A word of forewarning: Prepare yourself for some culinary surprises.

Additionally, at the end of this chapter, I have included my own special health drink. I call it "The Drink To Your Health."

Why Salads Are Important

Everyone needs salads. Of all the foodstuffs we should have on a daily basis, salads rank at the top. There is no substitute for salads, no better way to provide the body with the specific enzymes, minerals, and vitamins found in them.

Depending on the ingredients used, there can be as many as seven vital reasons for eating salads:

1. Salads introduce <u>life force</u> into the body because they are made from raw foods, direct from the earth. Most salad ingredients are consumed in a completely natural, unadulterated state.
2. Salads give us chlorophyl, which in turn promotes ventilation of body pores, enabling the body to acquire oxygen better.
3. Salads give us iron, which enhances the production of hemoglobin.
4. Salads contain cellulose, which in turn promotes the peristaltic action necessary to food movement and elimination. In common terminology, salads provide "roughage."
5. Salads containing onions provide us with <u>aldehyde</u>, a natural antiseptic.
6. Salads containing <u>green</u> onion roots provide us with <u>auxins</u> (a type of hormone which especially aids the reproductivity of hair, as well as the genetic quality of hair passed on to one's descendants.
7. Salads contain enzymes which have the potential for slowing the aging process.

The Great Upside-down Salad

I have found a way to make a vegetable salad that everyone can enjoy eating, even people with

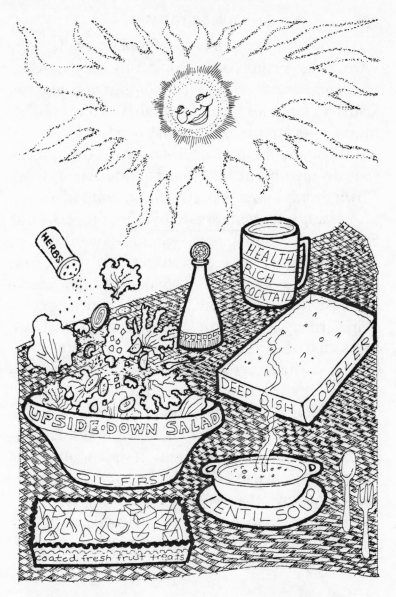

Prepare yourself for
some culinary surprises

ulcers or sensitive stomachs. Properly made, following the method outlined in this chapter, this salad can become one of the highlights of the meal. Usually, when a vegetable salad is prepared, the ingredients are placed into the bowl and a dressing is poured on, more or less in one concentrated spot. In my unique way of preparing the Upside-Down Salad, I always begin with the oil.

Using only cold-pressed oil (Sesame Seed Oil, Safflower Oil, Sunflower Seed Oil—any oil which has not had heat generated into it), coat the bowl liberally and then add Romaine lettuce, water cress, parsley, tomato, etc., making sure each piece is in turn coated with the oil. This simple act ensures that the next ingredients, the herbs, will adhere to the leaves and thus make the salad uniformly tasteful. The virtue of the Great Upside-Down Salad, then, is that it starts with the dressing.

Next add a variety (to taste) of herbs. Here I recommend herb seasonings such as oregano, thyme, basil, marjoram, dill, cayenne, curry, rosemary, and any other natural herbs favored.

OR, begin with a blend of both oil and herbs.

Remember always, that canned vegetables are dead food, and must not be used.

For Those with Special Chewing Problems

The procedure I have just described can be slightly altered for those with dental problems.

Because it is important that everyone eat one or two salads every day, I make this suggestion:

Put everything desired into an electric blender (starting with the tomato, for liquid content, and the oil, and even an optional raw egg, to taste), and grind together with remaining vegetables.

Vegetables

The list of vegetables used in the salad can be very extensive. The area where you live can determine what variety is available to you.

If possible, obtain fresh, deeply-colored vegetables. A good rule is to pick the green vegetable while it is dark green; the red when dark red; the yellow when a bright yellow. The deep colors in contrast to the pale colors usually indicate a perfect vegetable with high nutritive value.

If you care to make yours more hearty, or even into a complete meal, try adding hard-boiled eggs, shrimp, meats, chicken, etc. Pignolias (pine nuts) can be a pleasurable touch. A Julienne Salad with nuts and fruits can be a welcome change, but remember we get more vitamins and minerals from raw vegetables than from fruit.

Things To Remember about Salads

Never use old vegetables, canned vegetables, and never cook vegetables. Always mix them first with oil and herbs, and then, always remember to finish your meal with a full glass (8 ounces or more) of whole milk. This will aid in the full capturing of the chlorophyll and iron in the fresh vegetables.

But most important, don't forget those herbs! Herbs and oil go together just as naturally as girls and diamonds.

SALAD

The Great Upside-down Salad

You will need:

High quality cold-pressed oil, three tablespoons
Lettuce (green varieties are best), 1 head
Parsley, ½ bunch
Water cress, ½ bunch
Cucumbers or raw zucchini squash, 1
Carrots, 2
Celery, 6 stalks
Tomatoes, 3 large
Green onions (white roots and all), 4
Red Spanish onion, ½
Radishes, ½ bunch

1 tsp. of herb seasonings (Experiment with your own taste
   buds—use some or all)
Oregano
Sweet Basil
Black Pepper
Cayenne Pepper
Thyme
Marjoram
Dill
Curry
And others you may choose
Fresh crushed garlic (optional), 1 clove
Lemon juice or apple cider vinegar (optional), 2 tbsps.

Coat the bowl with the oil (or oil/herb mixture).

Break or cut the vegetables into bite size.

Put in the leafy vegetables first, including lettuce, parsley, and water cress. Toss and frost-coat with dressing.

Add remaining vegetables. Toss and mix well.

If desired, add fresh lemon juice or apple cider vinegar.

Mix thoroughly.

For greater vitamin and mineral content and for more flavors you can add fresh, raw corn, cut off the kernel; fresh, raw cauliflower; broccoli, spinach; cabbage; kale; or raw mushrooms.

Salt

I do not recommend the use of a lot of salt. The taste for salt is learned, therefore, it can also be unlearned. The seaweed, kelp, can be bought in powdered form at health food stores. Kelp contains the salt from the ocean as well as an important mineral we need, iodine. Try using this instead of commercial salt.

SALAD DRESSING

Here is a homemade salad dressing you might like to try as an alternate to the oil and herb mixture used in the Upside-Down Salad. You will need the following:

Tomatoes, 2 or 3
Cold-pressed oil, ⅔ cup
Fresh lemon juice or apple cider vinegar, ¼ cup
Fresh or dried dill, 1 tsp.
Garlic, 1 clove
Avocado, 1 (medium)
Cayenne pepper, sprinkling
Onion, 1
Sweet red or green pepper, 1
Egg, 1 (raw)
Powdered kelp or sea salt
Assorted herbs (oregano, basil, thyme, etc.)

Liquify these ingredients in a blender. Keep refrigerated in an airtight jar.

Basic Mayonnaise

Egg, 1
Lemon juice 2 tbsps. (fresh)
Honey, 1 tsp.
Powdered kelp or sea salt, ½ tsp.
Cayenne, sprinkling
Cold-pressed oil, 1 cup

Place all the ingredients in a blender (except the oil) and beat until thickened. Then add the oil and beat again thoroughly. Keep this mayonnaise refrigerated, and covered. You can be creative, using this recipe as a base. Add vinegar to make tart, fresh tomatoes to make Russian Dressing, chili to make hot, etc.

Basic Tomato Sauce

One large Onion, 1 (large, chopped)
Green pepper, 1 (small, chopped)
Tomatoes, 2 or 3 (cut)
Cold-pressed oil, 2 or 3 tbsps.
Powdered kelp or sea salt, ½ tsp.

Try adding herbs, but limit their use to about half a teaspoon (each). You might experiment with sweet basil, paprika, cayenne pepper, dill, rosemary, oregano, chili powder, majoram, etc.

Proceed as follows:

Lightly saute the onion in the oil.

Add tomtaoes and green pepper.

Season to taste with herbs and powdered kelp.

Cover the pot and simmer on a low flame for fifteen minutes, or until the vegetables are tender.

For a sauce with more body, add one cup of boiling water together with one tablespoon of arrowroot starch.

For variations, substitute some of the following: Mushrooms, fresh or dried dill, sorrel leaves, celery, small white onions, parsley, or cut okra.

Tangy Cheese Sauce

Butter, 1½ tbsps.
Powdered kelp, sea salt, or vegetable salt, sprinkling
Cayenne pepper, sprinkling
Milk, ¾ cup
Cheese (grated natural Cheddar, Swiss, or Jack), ¾ cup

Melt the butter on a low flame. Sprinkle in the seasonings. Pour in the milk, and mix well. Cook until well-heated, but do not boil. Add the cheese, and stir.

SOUPS

Most families in America no longer take the time to make homemade soups. What a pity! The nourishment of homemade soup is far superior to any found in cans.

Lentil Soup

Lentils (soaked overnight in two cups of water), 2 cups
Onion, 2 (chopped)
Milk (room temperature), 2 cups
Garlic (mashed), 1 clove
Carrots (chopped), 2 or 3
Celery (including the tops), 4 stalks
Green pepper (two, chopped)
Cold-pressed oil, 2 tbsps.
Parsnip (chopped), 1
Vegetable broth powder, ⅓ cup
Assorted herbs (kelp, bay leaf, or sage)

Sauté the onions in the oil. Add the lentils together with the water used for soaking. Cook for 1½ hours. Add the remaining vegetables, broth powder seasoning, and cook for one more hour. Just before serving, add room temperature milk to the hot soup and stir well.

Vegetable Soup

Tomatoes (4, cut)
Cabbage (2 cups, chopped—Savoy cabbage, if available)
Carrots (2 or 3, diced)
Celery (chop 6 stalks, including the tops)
Parsley (1 bunch, chopped)
Onion (2, chopped)
Parsnip (2, diced)
Green pepper (1, chopped)
Lima beans (1 cup)
String beans (1 cup, chopped)
Vegetable broth powder (½ cup)
Kelp and assorted herb seasonings
Water (2 cups)

Heat the water and add all the vegetables, broth powder, and seasonings. Bring to a boil. Cook for 30 minutes, or until the vegetables are tender.

Mung Bean Soup

Mung beans are of the soybean family, and are one of the best sources of protein. (Chinese bean sprouts come from mung beans.) Mung

Bean Soup is an excellent variety to have in one's cuisine. One advantage is that it only requires 1 hour to make. (Soybeans, in comparison, require 4–6 hours.)

Mung beans, 2 cups
Water (boiled), 4 cups
Onion (chopped), 2
Cold-pressed oil, 3 tbsps.
Carrots (diced), 2
Parsnip (diced), 2
Celery (diced, including the tops), 6 stalks
Vegetable broth powder, 3 tbsps.
Powdered kelp or sea salt, ½ tsp.
Assorted herbs, sprinkling

Sauté the onions in the oil until tender. Pour in the boiling water, then the mung beans. Cook for 15 minutes. Add the remaining ingredients, and cook for 45 minutes longer.

The "Almost-Raw" Soup

Your electric blender can help you make a nutritious, "almost-raw" soup.

Fresh peas (shelled), 1 cup
Corn (cut from the cob), 1 cup
Celery (diced), 1 cup
Banana squash (diced), 1 cup
Zucchini squash (sliced), 1 cup
Green onions (chopped), 6
Powdered kelp, ½ tsp.
Sweet basil and paprika, dash
Milk, 3 cups

Liquify all ingredients, including the milk, in a blender. Remove to pot. Heat without boiling. Add a pat of butter to each bowl when served.

DESSERTS

Plain fresh raw fruit is a fine dessert, but there are times when you want to enjoy eating something special.

Here are some suggestions for exciting homemade desserts that need no cooking or baking.

Fruit Surprise

For this dessert you can try different combinations, creating new inter-blended flavors.

Optional Fresh Fruits	Optional Berries
Persimmons	Blueberries
Bananas	Raspberries
Apples	Strawberries
Pears	Boysenberries
Melons	
Oranges	
Tangerines	
Peaches	
Apricots	

You will need:

Selected fruit (prepare as for a pie, either peeled, cut fine, mashed, or left whole), 2 cups
Date sugar, ⅓ cup
Lemon juice (fresh), 1 tsp.
Heavy cream (whipped), 2 cups
  OR
Yogurt, 1½ cups

Spoon the lemon juice into the prepared fruit. Gently work the date sugar through the fruit. Fold in the whipped cream or yogurt. Carefully spoon mixture into a bowl or into individual dessert glasses. Add coconut or nuts (finely grated, sprinkled on top). Refrigerate at least one hour before serving.

Deep-dish, Raw-apple Cobbler

Tart apples, 3
Fresh lemon juice, 3 tbsps.
Honey, ½ cup
Heavy sweet cream or yogurt, ¼ cup
Cinnamon, ½ tsp.
Wheat germ, 1 tbsp.
Sesame seeds (toasted and ground), ¼ cup
Almond butter, 3 tbsps.
Almonds (crushed), 1½ cups

Mix the almond butter with the crushed almonds, and blend thoroughly. Pack down into a bowl, and set aside. Combine the wheat germ, sesame seeds, cinnamon, and mix well. Let stand.

Grate apples coarsely or slice very thin. Coat the apples well with the lemon juice. Pour in the honey, and fold in the sweet cream or yogurt.

Now, stir the combination of wheat germ, sesame seeds, and cinnamon throughout the apple mixture. Spread the prepared almonds over the top. Keep refrigerated for at least two hours.

Coated Fresh Fruit Treats

Pineapple (cut in 2-inch squares)
Grapefruit sections (each segment cut into 2 or 3 pieces)
Melon, in season (cut in 2-inch squares)
Honey, 1 cup

Combine one cup of the following: Wheat germ, sunflower seed meal, toasted sesame seeds, powdered carob, and coconut flakes.

Blend all dry ingredients and let stand in a wide bowl. Insert a toothpick in each piece of fruit and roll immediately first in the bowl of honey, then in the bowl of dry ingredients.

Serve at room temperature or chilled.

Next we come to a powerhouse surprise—a fantastic skin and body builder.

The Drink To Build Your Health

Beneficial guidelines, to help you tackle skin problems, are presented throughout the book. To top everything, here is an added boost to hasten skin health.

The ingredients I have combined for a "food-drink" have unlimited potential to step up recovery and make good results appear much sooner. Also, overall body energy can be increased. This drink is charged with rich enzymes and live germinating food. It is excellent as a complete breakfast or lunch.

Miracle-energy Drink

This recipe was created by a famous physician who was dedicated to the task of fulfilling all the nutritive needs of the body. The wonder of this drink is that it will keep you looking young. Also, after faithfully partaking of the MIRACLE-ENERGY DRINK for about six months, you will be amazed to find that your energy level has increased noticeably. This drink provides complete nutrition, taken either as breakfast or lunch.

Into a blender, place two teaspoons of chia seeds. Pulverize.
Add:

Raw certified or homogenized milk, 2 cups
Eggs (raw), 4
Wheat germ oil, 2 tsps.
Quality cold-pressed oil, 2 tsps.
Powdered organic calcium or bone-meal powder, 2 tsps.
Brewer's yeast, 1 tbsp.
Kelp powder, ½ tsp.
Rose hips powder, 1 tsp.
Raw wheat germ, 4 tbsp.
Banana, 1

Blend well together.
Fresh fruit may be added, either coconut, apple, papaya, or berries.
If the mixture is too thick, add a little milk.

Keep refrigerated at all times. Eight ounces of this drink is a complete meal.

The foregoing menus, recipes, and special lists of foodstuffs were designed for (1) nutritive value, (2) dietary balance, and (3) vitamin and mineral content.

Sometimes, though we try hard and make good plans, our diet does not contain all the vitamins and minerals we need.

The next chapter is about this subject and deserves your close attention.

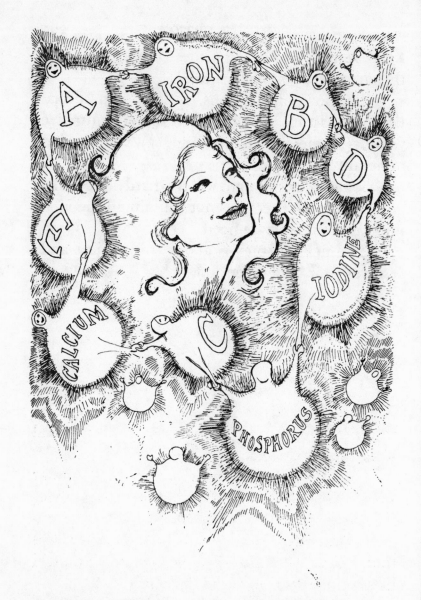

Play safe—round out your nutrition with supplements

16.

Do you really need vitamins and minerals?

Over the years, people have come to me after my lectures to discuss vitamins and minerals. They have spoken of their earnest investigation into the subject, trying to learn if there is a real necessity for these supplements.

Many of these people have told a similar story. When they asked their doctors for advice regarding vitamins, they were given empty answers rather than hard facts. Most often, they were told, "They won't do you any harm, so if you feel like taking them, go ahead."

It is to the credit of many that they did try vitamins and they did notice the difference. They became "do-it-yourself' health watchers, to their benefit.

207

Vitamins deserve more attention than they have received; minerals also. These natural accessory factors (which is what vitamins were first called) play a leading role in good health. And good health is the only promulgator of healthy skin.

A Brief History of Vitamins

Vitamin C made the first and most dramatic entrance upon the stage of science long before the word vitamin was even coined.

For centuries, scurvy had been the plague of sailors at sea. In the 1600s, Admiral Sir Richard Hawkins searched frantically for a cure to this dread disease. By chance, he tried oranges and then lemons (at that time called limes in England) as a cure. But, sadly, when Sir Richard died in 1622, this hard-won information died with him.

One hundred and fifty years later, Dr. James Lind rediscovered these citrus fruits as preventives of scurvy, although his theory was poorly received by fellow physicians. But, in the end, fifty years later, enough convincing evidence had been accumulated to open their eyes. In time, English sailors even became known as "limeys," because of the lime juice given them while at sea.

In 1881, a phrase was adopted that described

vitamins quite aptly . . . "small quantities of substances essential to life." In 1911, Casmir Funk, a young Polish-born biochemist, developed what later became known as the "vitamin hypothesis." He stated that specific nutritional deficiencies were the cause of rickets, beriberi, scurvy, and pellagra. Finally, in 1913, after further work by Funk and others, it became established that "accessory factors" really did exist, and that a descriptive name was needed for them. That name was *vitamin,* from *vita* (Latin, *life*).

Funk's work continues today, if in the hands of others. In the intervening half-century, a great literature has sprung up about vitamins and much has been discovered. But this does not mean we know all we must. There is overwhelming evidence to indicate vitamin research has not nearly been concluded. But even so, we do know that vitamins are necessary to good health.

Vitamin Decline in Today's Foods

Drs. E. Cheraskin and W. M. Ringsdorf, Jr., have researched the effects of vitamins on health and disease. They cite a Department of Health, Education, and Welfare study, published in 1960, which revealed that there has been a steady decline in vitamin content available from food.

A goodly proportion of produce reaching our markets is nutritionally poor. This is largely owing to the attitude of farmers. Enormous crops are today's goal, and chemical fertilizers—developed with emphasis on fast growth—are used to achieve this. The result is a vitamin- and mineral-deficient soil which yields vitamin- and mineral-deficient crops.

Cheraskin and Ringsdorf went on to show that the overcooking of food can bring the loss of natural vitamins and minerals to as much as 90 percent.

Are you one of those who devitalizes your food by overcooking, thereby dangerously toying with the health in your body?

Vitamin Destroyers

Up to now, we have been discussing agricultural and kitchen blunders which result in vitamin loss. But there are other powerful, insidious foes that literally steal vitamins from our very bodies. There are many such enemies.

Some of them are:

1. **Coffee is a drain on the Vitamin B supply in our bodies.**
2. **Smoking destroys Vitamin C (this is a loss**

which cannot be fully compensated for with Vitamin C tablets).

3. Alcoholic beverages make demands on the body's Vitamin B supply.

4. Artificial sweets drain B vitamins from the body.

5. Chlorine in drinking water destroys Vitamin E. Chlorine dioxide (used in bread) and rancid oils or inferior fats also destroy Vitamin E.

6. Fluorides destroy enzyme phosphatase, a catalyst which enhances vitamin efficiency.

7. Vitamins B and C, being water soluble, are constantly washed out of the body, and therefore require constant replenishment.

8. Chemical additives in prepared foods have a tendency to smother vitamins.

9. Air pollution plays a devastating role in our lives. Common pollutants have a tendency to shroud the effectiveness of all vitamins.

Another critical loss of vitamins and minerals results from drug use. Hoffman-La Roche, Ltd. of New Jersey, a large drug firm, deals with this in their publication, *Vitamins in the Treatment of Toxic Manifestations and Side Effects of Drugs.* In this work, it is made clear that drugs can create an abnormal loss of essential vitamins. Such an innocuous drug as the common antibiotic can strip the digestive tract of friendly bacteria. More and more, it is being found that massive doses of antibiotics must be offset by corrective measures. Yogurt and acidophilus are used to restock the colon with necessary protective bacteria.

What Do Vitamins Do for You?

Vitamins act as body-sparkplugs when they join chemically with oxygen, enzymes, minerals, and hormones. In so doing, they create other necessary chemical compounds. It might be said these supplements give us the "steam" to ride smoothly on life's track.

However, each of our dietary requirements is different. The uniqueness of our fingerprints, as an example, is nothing compared to our systemic uniqueness. That is why we can only offer general suggestions. The required fine-tuning is the individual's responsibility.

Individual Needs

Professor Frederick B. Hutt, a Cornell University geneticist specializing in poultry husbandry, found that genetic differences in domestic fowl created variations in vitamin and mineral requirements. These individualities, he states, are inborn and cause variances in the host-body's ability to synthesize enzymes. These variances, in turn, can be balanced out with vitamin and mineral supplements.

That a human parallel to this equation exists has been authenticated by biologists. Dr. Roger Williams, University of Texas professor of biochemistry, in his book, *Biochemical Individuality,* draws such a conclusion.

An Overview of Vitamins

There are many fine vitamin texts. These books, ranging from general reading to ponderous tomes, are easily available and I suggest that the interested reader refer to them. The subject is touched upon only lightly here.

Suffice it to say vitamins can be an added perimeter of defense around the fortress which defends us from the enemy—bad health. But this does not mean they can stand alone, or that we can survive on a diet of vitamins. They are referred to as supplements because they are exactly that.

Vitamin researchers have identified from fifteen to seventeen vitamins to date (depending on whom we believe) and think there may be many more. Following is a list of those vitamins most pertinent to our text.

Vitamin A

Vitamin A is found in foods deriving from both plants and animals. From plants, we receive Vitamin A in "carotene" form. When we consume it, our body has first to convert the carotene into Vitamin A. The animal source is probably better because the conversion has already been made.

Cod Liver Oil, as stated, is one of the primary sources of Vitamin A.

Our skin, mucous membranes, eyes, circulatory system, and joints are only a few of the many areas of the body which demand Vitamin A. Of these, the skin's need for Vitamin A is probably best known.

Also, Vitamin A is known to lower the blood-cholesterol level.

Vitamin B

"Vitamin B" is not one but a group of single, important vitamins which collectively are known

as the "B-complex." Although each of these vitamins has a special function, the B-complex works
harmoniously as a whole, and that is how we refer
to it here.

Most people are unaware that Vitamin B is
as important to skin care as is Vitamin A. In fact,
the skin—when healthy—is the principle storehouse of Vitamin B.

If you are unaccountably fatigued or irrita-
ble, there is a strong possibility your body is de-
ficient of B vitamins. They are necessary for nerve
well-being, and they are especially necessary for
coping with the stress of daily living.

B vitamins, because they are water-soluble,
cannot be long-retained in the body and therefore
must be replenished continually.

Vitamin C

Vitamin C has been called the "master vitamin." It is basic to health and life, and the body
must have it to function. Principally, Vitamin C
is a purveyor of hydrogen, an essential substance
in the burning of our foodstuffs. Additionally,
Vitamin C is important as a connective tissue
bond.

The human body has lost the capability to
manufacture its own Vitamin C. We need it every

day—preferably from natural foods, but from supplements, if necessary.

There is no danger of getting too much Vitamin C—the body will throw off any excess it cannot use.

Vitamin D

This has been called the "sunshine vitamin." Most often, it is produced by the skin when there is contact with the sun.

The pivotal role of Vitamin D lies in its ability to promote properly the absorption of calcium and phosphorus by the body. Additionally, Vitamin D is important for correct bone and teeth structuring, for healthy fingernails, etc.

Vitamin E

Vitamin E, although a relative newcomer, has been researched for many years in many laboratories. Findings have borne out much that pioneers suspected at the outset.

Two of these pioneers, Drs. Evan and Wilfrid Shute of Ontario, Canada, concluded that Vitamin E is of central importance to the cardiovascular system. Others later believed this vitamin improved fertility. Of greater moment, and higher agreement, Vitamin E has proven miraculous in the healing of wounds and burns.

The reported attributes of Vitamin E go on to make an impressive list.

Vitamin F

This vitamin forms the fatty protein known as myelin, which sheathes the major nerves of the body, including the spinal cord. A serious lacking of Vitamin F can give rise to mental disorders, and possibly even multiple sclerosis. As I have stated previously, Vitamin F is readily available in Cod Liver Oil.

Vitamin K

This is another of the lesser-known vitamins. This is probably so because it is not available in supplement form without a doctor's prescription.

Vitamin K is the blood-clotting vitamin, and essential to the body. It is found naturally in leafy greens, which makes them mandatory in our diets.

Minerals

Following is a list of minerals which our bodies—in some degree—require.

CALCIUM: The bone-building mineral. Also helps sustain a rhythmic heart. Adds to one's vitality and endurance.

COPPER: Assists the body to absorb and utilize iron. Increases the formation of red blood cells.

COBALT: Stimulates the appetite and production of red blood cells.

IRON: Carries oxygen to the blood, and is required in the manufacture of hemoglobin.

FLUORINE: Reduces the occurrence of dental caries.

MANGANESE: Activates the enzymes and other minerals in your system.

MAGNESIUM: Helps to maintain normal functioning of both your nerves and muscles.

MOLYBDENUM: Necessary for carbohydrate metabolism.

PHOSPHORUS: Also valuable for better bone and teeth structure.

POTASSIUM: Promotes normal heart action, controls nervousness, and establishes better muscle tone.

SULPHUR: An essential mineral for good skin, hair, and fingernails.

ZINC: An aid to normal tissue function, especially nervous (brain) tissue. (Recall the old saw "You've got to have zinc to think.") Also utilized in protein and carbohydrate metabolism.

Reasons Vitamins and Minerals Are an Aid to Nutrition

The soils from which our foods derive are becoming depleted of nature's nutrients. Moreover, because of commercial considerations, produce is usually harvested either too late or too soon and shipped to market. Next, these are treated to give added store-life.

When these products reach our kitchen, cooking is the final insult which robs them of minerals and vitamins.

For all these reasons, and more, you owe it to yourself to round out each day's diet with adequate supplements.

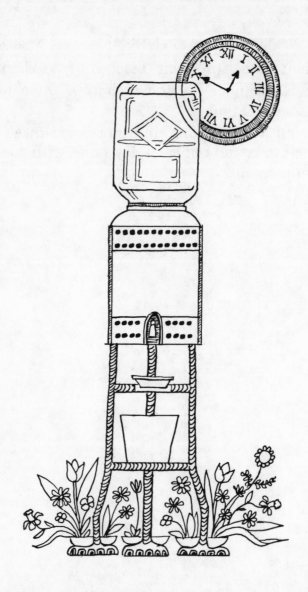

Life cannot exist without
water
but know when to drink it

Water...
How important
is it to your skin?

Throughout this book, great emphasis is placed upon the incompatibility of water and oil. The object has been to make you aware that water plays an important role in the assimilation of your food . . . and therefore is critical to skin health.

Life, of course, cannot exist without water. But even though it is vital, it is also usually abundant, and so many of us have come to take it for granted. This is unfortunate, because there is much we should know about water. Indeed, the subject warrants close and special attention.

The Miracles and Wonders of Water

Miracles have been attributed to natural springs. Millions of religiously inspired people have made the holy trek to Lourdes, France, and to other similar springs reknowned for their healing capability. In our own country, we have seen headlines about the unusually strong, cavity-free teeth of the inhabitants in Deaf Smith County, Texas. This has been credited to an abundance of natural fluorides in the water.

Hot mineral spas throughout the world have helped soothe throngs of people troubled with aches and pains.

In Hunzaland, Tibet, the life span reaches one hundred twenty years and more. Reproductive capabilities continue on to advanced years. The simplicity of life, the clean air, and the unadulterated foods eaten are cited as reasons for this. But, more than these things, it is believed one of the outstanding features is the water. It is not sparkling clear, but instead slightly murky. Supposedly it contains special life-giving minerals.

These are but a few accounts of the wonderwork of water.

What You Should Know about Water

The leading source of drinking water is rain. Underground water, as well as that from springs, streams, and lakes, all come from rain. It is all fresh water with the exception of ocean water, which is saline. Sea water contains all the minerals that have streamed down from the mountains. These minerals accumulate in the ocean and become concentrated through an endless process of evaporation. Clouds are formed from the evaporated mineral-free water. Eventually, soft-water rain comes showering from these clouds.

The mineral content of natural water is geographically determined. This is why some water is hard, some soft, and some even toxic.

Natural disasters such as floods, earthquakes, tornadoes, and plagues usually produce dangerously polluted water. Accompanying the enormity of devastation is a loss of sanitary conditions.

Today, with human waste and chemical contaminates from industry and agriculture all too often infiltrating our public water systems, we have pollution. To make the water safe, chlorine is added to destroy bacteria.

Many consider drinking chlorine, even in minute amounts, a health hazard. This has led to a search for unchlorinated water. The result has been availability of a variety of types of water specifically offered as an improvement over chlorinated water. But these have provoked uncompromising disagreement over which is the most healthful to drink. Much has been written and said to present the different points of view.

The Controversy about Water

Which do you drink, distilled water (hypotonic), mineral-bearing water (hypertonic), water that has synthetic fluoride added to it, or water that comes out of the tap (isotonic)?

The first, distilled, has all minerals and life force out of it. Exponents of distilled water say that undistilled water contains much dangerous matter along with its beneficial minerals: radiation fallout, pollution, etc. They argue that these minerals can be replaced safely through the consumption of fruits and vegetables, wholesome foods, or mineral supplements.

Advocates of mineral-rich water feel strongly about their convictions. In addition, they stress that distilled water leeches natural minerals already in the body. They see such a situation as a serious threat.

When the story about Deaf Smith County reached public attention, a drive was made in some parts of the country to add synthetic fluoride to water systems. This procedure has been adopted in some cities. Further, fluoridation has become a nationwide political issue because of concern that synthetic fluoride may be more of a detriment than a benefit to health.

Some people choose to have man-made soft water in their homes. This is achieved by the addition of equipment which treats the water with salt. But the increased quantity of sodium in water, if it is consumed regularly, may prove harmful to the body.

My Thoughts On Drinking Water

For drinking, I feel bottled spring water should be the choice. It must be noncarbonated. I mention this because of the many naturally carbonated waters which are sold on the market. These waters, though naturally carbonated, are still unhealthy. They are charged with gases which the body cannot fully discharge. Residue from the carbonation remains in the body and creates damage—especially to the skin.

My primary concern, as I have said elsewhere in the book, centers mainly on the proper time and temperature of water when it is drunk.

Here again I want to stress that coffee, tea,

lemonade, etc., are all "treated" water. Any oil-free liquid is in the same class as water and must be respected for its incompatibility with oil or any oil-bearing food.

How Much Water Do We Require?

The average adult male body carries about 100 pounds of water. This liquid forms about 70 percent of the body. Blood is 90 percent water, bones are 22 percent water. Every cell contains water.

In survival emergencies, one can live longer without food than without water. If there is as little as 20 percent water-loss in the body, it can mean dehydration and death.

A healthy balance can be maintained by consuming one centimeter of liquid for each calorie of food. This is the equivalent of eight glasses of liquid with 2000 calories of food. "Liquid" does not necessarily mean "water." Sources of liquid can be found in milk, soup, fruits and vegetables, etc. As a matter of fact, all foods have some liquid in varying degrees.

Milk, for example, is 87 percent water, and even such unlikely items as peanuts and coffee beans have small quantities of it. I have prepared a special chart below, showing the percentage of water in various foods.

Foods	Percentage of Water
Egg	74.0
Cottage Cheese	74.0
Cream Cheese	53.3
Cheddar Cheese	39.0
Butter	15.5
Veal	71.0
Liver	70.9
Chicken	67.1
Round Steak	67.0
Lamb	66.0
Chuck Roast	65.0
Frankfurters	64.3
Corned Beef	57.0
Ham	53.0
Spareribs	53.0
Pork	50.0
Oysters	87.1
Codfish	82.6
Salmon	67.4
Tuna	57.7
Sardines	47.0
Cucumbers	96.1
Squash	95.0
Lettuce	94.8
Tomatoes	94.1
Celery	93.7
Radishes	93.6
Asparagus	93.0
Spinach	92.7
Cabbage	92.4
Cauliflower	91.7
Broccoli	89.7
Carrots	88.2
Onions	87.5
Potatoes	77.8
Green Peas	74.3
Cantaloupe	94.0
Watermelon	92.1
Oranges	87.2
Peaches	86.9
Apples	84.1
Pears	82.7
Bananas	74.8
Whole Wheat Bread	39.7
Rye Bread	37.6
Cake	26.8
Oatmeal	8.3
Cashews	3.5
Walnuts	3.3
Almonds	3.2
Peanut Butter	1.9
Yeast, Bakers	70.9
Yeast, Brewers	7.0
Wheat Germ	11.0

As you can see, there is some water in everything we eat. We can rely on this as part of our daily liquid requirement.

Many people find that three glasses of water a day, taken in advance of meals, prove satisfactory. There are circumstances where more is wanted—such as in the summer or following great exertion. When perspiring, water must be replenished.

Then, too, spicy, salty, or too much sweet foods provoke an increased desire for liquids. In such instances, beware. Excessive fluid retention can waterlog the body. Most overweight people are victims of this indulgence.

Occasional violation of good health rules will not cause any serious damage. But regular bad habits must be examined, and changed. The price of indulgence is always too steep.

We can drink all the water we desire, but we must at the same time respect the correct timing and temperature rules, as well as sensible standards of nutrition.

Quenching parched cravings with iced and/or "treated" water at mealtimes can leave you with a parched skin. If you do this, your skin will be shortchanged and denied the lubrication and moisturization it desperately requires. I have thoroughly explained this process in chapters eleven and thirteen.

Your body, as a general rule, decides for itself how much water it needs every day.

Be Water-wise

Following are the six basic guidelines which should govern your intake of water:

1. **Never drink water with meals. Restrict water intake to 10 minutes prior to meals or until 3 hours after meals.**
2. **Be wary of camouflaged water. Coffee, tea, lemonade, punch, soft drinks, alcoholic beverages, etc., are all essentially water and are governed by #1 above.**
3. **Avoid all carbonated water.**
4. **Avoid iced drinks. The ice-cube is one of the most dangerous inventions of man.**
5. **Drink one or two glasses of room temperature water upon arising. This is a very good method of flushing the kidneys.**
6. **Never add water to milk.**

Water, at first thought, seems to be universal, benign, tasteless, colorless, and plentiful beyond description. But not all of these characteristics hold. Particularly, it is not benign. Under certain circumstances, it can do more harm than good. Water, like fire, can be both useful and destructive, and for this reason, you owe it to yourself to make certain you do not misuse it.

Water, for the most part a simple, necessary, nondangerous element, is very much a part of our lives by natural design.

However, some things have become a part of our life despite natural design. One of these is margarine, which is neither simple, necessary, nor without danger.

18

Why margarine is bad for your skin

About fifty years ago, a product called oleo-margarine found its way into this country from Europe. An imitation of butter, it was then used primarily for economic reasons, since it cost so much less than the real thing. Some persons welcomed this artificial butter, mistakenly believing it contained fewer calories.

During the past twenty-five years, another belief has evolved, that margarine is a dietary aid because of its low cholesterol content. This has happened because we have been touted into believing that cholesterol-bearing foods are bad for us.

The food advertising media have capitalized on this. We are constantly being barraged with praises for food products that are glorified because they are low in cholesterol. This has been interpreted by many to mean our bodies do not need cholesterol at all. In fact, we have been led to believe cholesterol is an archenemy of good health. As I have explained in chapter eleven, "Cholesterol and Your Skin," this is not true.

Even nature's butter is rich in cholesterol, and for this reason many people also regard it as a dietary taboo. Because of this kind of brainwashing, we have seen a vast increase in the use of margarine. In-depth research is now revealing the serious consequences of this shift from butter to margarine . . . on the skin as well as on the whole body.

How Margarine Originated

Margarine, like the jet airplane and the atomic bomb, came into existence because of a war. During last century's Franco-Prussian War, a butter shortage developed. Something had to be done. In 1869 some ingenious French monks managed to concoct a substitute for butter. They prepared it from suet, whale oil, and other animal fats. In time it became known as oleomargarine (*oleo* [Latin, *oil*] + *margarine* [from margaric acid]).

But, after the war, the dairy herds once again flourished and so the supply of butter was replenished. Only the poor continued to use the new product oleomargarine.

The Growth of Margarine in the United States

During the past fifty years, margarine has undergone a series of growths and changes.

Always trailing in the image of butter, the manufacturers have continually striven for the look and taste of the natural product. The stark whiteness of the original oleomargarine was unappealing to the eye. Attempts were made to duplicate the color of butter.

At this point, the dairy industry protested by trying to protect the integrity of butter, and, for a while, successfully kept margarine from being sold in an artificially precolored condition. Through state legislation, synthetic coloring was prohibited.

To combat this restriction, the producers of oleomargarine first offered gelatin-clad perles of food-coloring with each package. This could be blended into the oleo at home, if desired.

During the Depression thirties, this bogus butter was very widely used. Whether or not it was deserving, oleomargarine came to be considered a staple in most of our homes.

As the margarine industry grew, it was able,

through lobbyists and the like, gradually to overpower the dairy industry. In time, the artificial-coloring restriction was lifted.

Oleomargarine became a much-used food commodity, and, in time, the diminutive term "margarine" became adopted.

Today, margarine has become a common item in kitchens, so common, in fact, that a whole generation of young adults fail to realize it was originally a stopgap food substitute, brought into existence by desperation.

The Plastic Truth

The regulation formulated by the Department of Agriculture—and accepted as standard in many states—specifically defines oleomargarine (margarine) as ". . . the plastic food prepared with one or more (of the optional) fat ingredients."

The definition goes on to tell us these "optional ingredients" can be obtained from the following sources, either alone or combined: (1) cattle, sheep, hogs, or goats, (2) milk (cow's) or its products (creamy buttermilk, dry or condensed milk) , and (3) finely ground soybeans (whole or dehulled) . The fat content of the completed product must be at least 80 percent, the same as in butter.

Oleomargarine began as a money-saving item in the kitchen, but its commercial potential was finally seen and taken advantage of by opportunistic producers. This was brought about when the medical community advised an increase in the intake of polyunsaturated fatty acids and a simultaneous reduction of intake of saturated fatty acids.

Business barons, recognizing great financial possibilities, ordered a concentrated effort to develop margarine with a new look. It was an all-out campaign.

A dramatic change in the preparation of margarine took place. The big switch was from animal (saturated) fats to vegetable (polyunsaturated) fats. There are still some cheap brands of margarine which very quietly continue to use lard, or other animal fats, as a base ingredient.

These changes brought about a radical increase in the oleomargarine business, which in turn produced a flood of competitive margarines. A superabundance of commercials on TV and radio, plus ads in newspapers and magazines, resulted. These food barons were all vying for the same dollar.

What started out as simple mock butter, had turned into a mockery. So much attention had been paid to the capturing of the consumer that the quality of the product became secondary.

The Making of Modern Margarine

As mentioned, modern margarine is usually made from vegetable oils. These are extracted from a wide range of oil-rich plant sources, such as corn, safflower, soya beans, peanuts, cottonseeds, and red palms.

But the freshly extracted "crude" oil contains impurities. These include certain free fatty acids, mucilagenous substances, and resins. They need to be removed because they sometimes add unappealing colors, flavors, or odors to the final product.

Hence, processing. The oils undergo refining, bleaching, and deodorizing. Refining removes the free fatty acids. Bleaching is done with inert materials, such as clay, which strain out the matter responsible for the undesirable colors. Deodorization is achieved through steaming the oil under reduced pressure.

Old-fashioned oleomargarine, when made

from animal fat, was a simple, uncomplicated process. The animal fat—or tallow—was naturally disposed to remain solid (candles and soap are still made from animal tallow) .

Modern margarine has to be solidified by a process called hydrogenation. This is done with the aid of nickel, a result of which is that solid vegetable tallow is created. And, before it is finished, numerous other questionable ingredients are added. Among these can be found: fillers (such as dry milk solids, soya powders) ; flavorings and colorings (for enhancement) ; synthetic vitamins (supposedly for enrichment) ; preservatives (to prevent spoilage, ensuring longer shelf-life) .

The original oleomargarine was essentially a saturated fat, made of animal tallow. Now, of course, we know saturated fats can result in higher cholesterol levels and bring on heart problems, etc. Therefore, it would seem the modern margarines, especially those made of polyunsaturated fats, should be an improvement. But, actually, are they?

Margarine Research

Over the years, chemists and physicians have been trying to determine the overall physical effects of margarine. Often they have found it to be a questionable, highly suspect substance. From a vast body of available research literature, I have chosen three samples to illustrate my point.

In 1960, there occurred in the Netherlands an epidemic which ultimately became identified as the "Dutch Margarine Disease." Researchers later called it "The So-Called Margarine Disease."*

This very real disorder, with skin eruptions as its dominant symptom, began in western Germany in 1958. When it reached the Netherlands in 1960, it was first observed in Rotterdam by a general practitioner as being the result of a specific margarine. A study was conducted by the State Health Inspector and the special margarine was removed from markets.

The margarine in question had been "improved" to have a better taste and to be splatter-proof in the frying pan. A toxicological investigation showed that an emulgator had been added to effect this "improvement."

A second example has to do with the clotting of blood. Researchers at the Thrombosis Research Hospital of Oslo, Norway, concluded after exhaustive testing that normal butter has no effect on the clotting time of human blood. Margarine, on the

* Excerpted from: "The Epidemic of Polymorph Toxic Erythema in the Netherlands in 1960," by I. W. H. Mali and K. E. Malten.

other hand, produced a measurable acceleration of clotting time in the same control group.*

Our third example deals with chemical research into the physical nature of "fatty acids." Dr. Antoine Gattereau, assistant professor, University of Montreal, in an article on margarine appearing in the *Canadian Medical Association Journal,* August 1, 1970, states that during the hydrogenation process of the polyunsaturated oils, a peculiar transformation occurs. The oils that began as unsaturated fatty acids ("cis" isomers) became "trans" fatty acids. Evidence shows that "trans" fatty acids behave much more as saturated than unsaturated acids.

When certain producers learned of this, they quickly turned to marketing a margarine which was only "partially hydrogenated." These margarines are blends—some of the oil having been hydrogenated and some not. It is questionable to me whether this product is any less harmful than its companion products.

Another Myth about Margarine

Many heart patients, switched from butter to margarine and thereafter observing a lower cho-

* Excerpted from: "Blood Factor XI After Fat-Rich Meals," by O. Egeberg.

lesterol level, believe that margarine helped. But that is far too simplistic a conclusion. Much has to be observed and weighed to arrive at the true picture. Restrictions can include prohibitions of most fats, salt, fried foods, junk foods, as well as a weight-reduction program, all of which ordinarily results in a total change in that heart patient's way of life. In my opinion, the role attributed to margarine in the lowering of cholesterol is a myth.

Conclusion

Whereas in this chapter we have been addressing ourselves to margarine, we must not overlook the thrust of the whole book: skin care. The two are interrelated.

Margarine, under the very best of conditions is an unacceptable substitute for butter. To worsen this situation, most margarines are <u>not</u> produced under the best conditions. There are no standards to limit hydrogenation; in fact, there are virtually no controls whatever to watchdog the production of margarines. The result, of course, is that the way is clear for producers to concentrate on profit rather than product.

What we must understand is that margarine becomes a trans-fatty acid which the human body is not equipped to metabolize properly. Because of this, margarine—in the form of sebum—finds its way to the skin. There it surfaces and becomes a visible blandishment.

I find myself more and more impatient with the continuance of favorable propaganda bestowed upon margarine. It just doesn't deserve it.

The human body has a thousand ways to let us know something has gone wrong. Some of these symptoms deal directly with digestion.

The next chapter which deals with irregularity addresses this problem.

19.

Daily regularity ...A necessity for Healthier skin

In the pursuit of a healthy skin—the problem of irregularity must not be overlooked.

The rejuvenation or rebuilding process is of utmost importance for a youthful skin and body. Constipation can restrict this from happening.

When elimination is slowed down or stopped, stagnation can set in. This can lead to a chain of circumstances that deters good body functioning.

For some people, the one way to overcome irregularity is through laxatives.

Elimination . . . Not a Simple Problem

The dangerous effects of laxatives are being recognized more and more. The frequent use of

harsh cathartics can leave one susceptible to serious diseases graver than constipation. At the same
time, friendly bacteria are being purged out of
the alimentary tract.

How to Achieve Natural Elimination

Unless you maintain regularity and proper
bowel habits you can be certain that your skin
will suffer.

My answer is not to propose laxatives or pur-
gatives. There is one substance which can correct
intestinal problems. It is little known, so in this
chapter I want to reveal the complete story of its
origin and effectiveness.

The food substance is called acidophilus. It
is a concentrated lactobacillus culture, available
inexpensively in most health food stores and in
some supermarkets.

To understand the value of this substance,
let me trace its medical history for you.

The one man who pioneered the theory
which I support—regarding constipation—was
Eli Metchnikoff. He was deputy director of the
Pasteur Institute in Paris. He spent his lifetime as
a microbiologist trying to determine how to prevent aging in humans.

Metchnikoff worked with thousands of patients for more than thirty years. Many of them lived to an age of one hundred twenty years or more. How did they accomplish this remarkably good health? Their secret was acidophilus.

They added acidophilus curd to their milk. By keeping it in a warm place it became completely converted into curds and whey. They then drank the whey and ate all of the curd.

In those days, they had to consume at least a pint a day. Fortunately, modern food manufacturers have developed a way to concentrate acidophilus into bottled form. Now, a person needs only two or three tablespoonsful a day.

We have Metchnikoff to thank for making all of this possible. He said: "Acidophilus is the strongest of the lactobacilli and best able to survive passage through the high hydrochloric acid juices of the stomach into the intestines where it thrives, especially if there is lactose (milk sugar or sweet whey in the diet."

Special Note: Blend Your Acidophilus

My own research indicates that for best results you should combine the liquid acidophilus with whole milk and other foods.

Place six ounces of milk in a blender—along with a raw egg, and perhaps half a banana. As a mixture, the two tablespoonsful of acidophilus will then be more thoroughly utilized by your digestive tract.

The purpose of this entire process is to have your body build a supply of "friendly" bacteria. By that I mean, you will be creating lactobacilli. These are microorganisms which are bred in your intestinal flora.

Without this bacterial chain reaction, toxins cannot be prevented from forming. This can cause your skin to suffer and perhaps develop blemishes.

Another valuable weapon is to keep your diet well supplied with wholesome, nourishing foods. Especially raw vegetables. They have, for your skin, a cleansing effect.

I will now contribute my recommended list of foods. And, I will show their value to help control constipation.

I submit them, below, in the order of their effectiveness.

FOOD	WHY IT IS BENEFICIAL
1. Raw Wheat Germ	Can correct a Vitamin B deficiency.
2. Brewer's Yeast	Highest known source of natural Vitamin B-complex.
3. Onions (Raw)	Contains aldehydes, to kill harmful bacteria.
4. Scallions (Raw)	To strengthen mineral reserves.
5. Natural Bran	An excellent bulk-forming food.
6. Figs (Black, unsulphured)	Mild laxative, to promote peristalsis.

FOOD	WHY IT IS BENEFICIAL
7. Prunes	Slow acting, but safe for delicate systems.
8. Dried Fruits	Good source of magnesium and manganese.
9. Green Celery (Raw)	Supplies natural sodium and chlorine.
lo. Cabbage (Raw)	Bulk-forming.

In addition, to combat constipation, I also favor the following foods. Cucumbers, whole wheat toast, wheat germ flake cereal, apples, raw carrots, legumes, Romaine lettuce, raw cauliflower, raw spinach.

Remember these specific foods. Pay special attention to the first half of the list, because it contains the four "prime factors." They are the Vitamin B-complex elements, aldehydes to fight certain bacteria, mild laxatives to enhance peristalsis and bulk.

If you will follow the ideas—and the foods—which I have presented above you will have little to worry about concerning constipation. After a while you will be able to see positive results by just looking in your own mirror.

The "Hot Water with Lemon Juice" Habit

The drinking of hot water with lemon juice first thing in the morning for regularity has a drying effect on the skin. Drinking the hot water alone will accomplish the same purpose without hurting the skin.

As you can see, it is important not to ignore any problem of irregularity. But deal with it in the healthiest and most wholesome manner . . . as is recommended here.

Twenty Questions: A summary quiz on skin

I always give the audiences attending any lectures an opportunity to ask questions. Frequently, I hear the same queries . . . the same skin problems seem to affect people of all age groups, in big cities and in little towns. Thus it might be helpful to <u>you</u> if I give a brief résumé. Here are the answers to the twenty questions which I hear most often.

Q. What harm will come to my skin if I stay out in the sun too long?

A. If your diet doesn't contain nutritive oils and vitality factors, your skin <u>will</u> become parched and harsh-looking.

Q. Can the sun ever be beneficial to the skin?

A. Yes. If your diet includes the correct oils, minerals, vitamins, etc. If you follow a good diet, the sun (in moderate amounts) is beneficial. However, the skin is more vulnerable to the very hot rays of the sun—between 11:00 a.m. and 3:00 p.m.

If in doubt, do your sunning during those hours when the sun-rays are less penetrating.

Q. What causes the oily skin on my forehead and nose?

A. You are probably eating too many low-grade food oils, like oleomargarine. Any fried oil, ice cream, or hydrogenated peanut butter are also taboo for you.

Q. I have always had dry skin. I found that I had to put oil on my skin after I bathe, and on my face immediately after washing it. Will your Cod Liver Oil regimen solve my problem?

A. Yes. However, it may take nearly six months of persevering patience to correct this.

Q. I have read where an oily face is caused by a deficiency of Vitamin B-6. I started taking this vitamin about a year ago, and I still have an oily face. Why?

A. This condition of yours goes far beyond the need for Vitamin B-6. You are probably damaging your skin by ingesting too many sugary liquids.

Q. Why do I have dandruff? I was told it may be a psychological problem.

A. Wrong. Primarily, dandruff is the result of being on a heavy sweets diet (including too much candy and ice cream). This leads to a Vitamin B deficiency which, in turn, causes the scalp to shed. Try using more Vitamin B-complex foods. Wheat germ, Brewer's yeast, and broiled calves' liver would also help. But psychological disturbances play only a secondary role.

Q. How can I avoid the threat of skin cancer?

A. I suggest at least three major rules to observe: 1. The use of Cod Liver Oil to keep the iodine content high in your skin. 2. Do not drink acid-bearing liquids. 3. Keep away from sugary liquids, especially carbonated drinks.

Q. Can good nutrition erase scars from the face?

A. No. Scar tissue, from a burn or accident, is irreversible through food sources.

Q. What causes acne, and why is it on the increase?

A. For most people, acne starts with a badly chosen diet during their puberty years. Adulteration of foods is largely responsible for the current rise and prevalence.

Q. What is the best treatment for young children who have psoriasis?

A. All acid-bearing liquids must be deleted from the diet. Fried oily foods should also be eliminated. My suggested Cod Liver Oil program should be started immediately.

Q. Why do so many teen-agers have blackheads and pimples?

A. Blackheads are most often owing to the consumption of

fried or inferior oils. They (the oils) go through the liver and produce carbon "clinkers." Pimples generally indicate a flooding of the skin by the intake of too many sugary liquids.

Q. Can a child develop a skin allergy by drinking milk?

A. Yes. If the mother's diet—during pregnancy—contained skim milk, soft drinks, or frozen juices.

Q. Is it permissible to take your Cod Liver Oil Mini-Milkshake at 11:00 P.M.?

A. Perfectly fine. As long as it's on an empty stomach. I would prefer that you drink the Mini-Milkshake one hour before breakfast.

Q. If you are taking the Cod Liver Oil mixture to help normalize your skin, should the oil be kept in the refrigerator?

A. It needn't be. Cod Liver Oil has a tendency to "repeat" if it is consumed ice cold.

Q. How can I get rid of the "pebble-like" skin texture on my nose?

A. One way is to make sure that your diet has at least 75 percent raw food. Emphasis should be on large green salads, daily. No salt in your diet. Make sure your kidneys are working well.

Q. What effect do Vitamin E creams and ointments have when applied directly to the skin?

A. They have healing power, especially to scar tissue areas. They have proven beneficial on burns.

Q. What is the cause of these dark pigmented spots, which are on the back of my hands?

A. That is a symptom of Vitamin B-complex deficiency. This can be accompanied by serrations along the edges of the tongue. These spots are often referred to as "liver spots." It is possible that the liver is losing its war . . . owing to a preponderance of sweets.

Q. Is there anything I can do about dark skin under my eyes?

A. Once dark circles are formed beneath the eyes, generally they are permanent. However, sound nutrition and sound sleep will help. Improving your blood circulation—with the help of Vitamin C—will also contribute much to the repair process. You must also try Schiatzu (finger-pressure).

Q. For many years, I have had itchy ears. Is mine a nutritional problem?

A. Yes I recommend that you build up your supply of essential fatty acids. The itchiness reflects the fact that your body is demanding a better diet.

Q. I have a continuous rash on my chest. Why?

A. The chest area has a large concentration of sebaceous glands. These glands reflect dietary mistakes. Your chest is a part of

the body which perspires easily and rashes can originate in
this area.

The questions we have published here are a
mere sampling of the skin inquiries which seem
to be uppermost in the public's mind. As you may
know, I give more than fifty lectures in different
cities every year. Usually I appear on both radio
and television interview programs. They often
invite listeners to ask questions by telephone.

If your specific question has not been answered in the list above, when you next hear me
on a radio talk show, pick up your telephone and
call the station. It will be a pleasure for me to
speak with you personally . . . and I will help
you with your skin problem, if I can.

Part Five
NATURAL OUTER SKIN CARE

21

Tips on natural skin beauty care

"Beauty is skin deep" if manufactured with deftly applied cosmetic make-up. Healthy skin has a natural glow of beauty that is manufactured from within by deftly chosen nutrients.

However, there are gifts of nature . . . balms for the skin, that <u>can</u> heal and <u>comfort</u> the skin.

Nature's Emollients for Skin

There are many natural potions and lotions made at home, including cucumber creams, strawberry masks, and other luscious-sounding concoctions. The stomach can properly digest these foods, but your outer skin cannot. These mixtures usually are suitable for soothing and pampering the skin.

While on my lecture tours, in different parts of the world, I have learned of emollients that come from plants, from the bark of trees, from fruits, from wonderful Nature. These healing and soothing balms are available to us if we would but seek them out.

ALOE VERA GEL

One of the finest is a gel that comes out of the Aloe Vera plant. This is a cactus plant well known in Indian folklore. It grows in dry and more arid climates. The thick green leaves of the plant hold this gel which heals burns, cuts, abrasions of the skin and, amazingly, with less than the usual amount of scarring. The healing of stomach ulcers have also been credited to the aloe vera gel, when consumed internally.

Aloe vera gel is excellent as a sunburn preventive.

This plant can be raised in the home or, if the climate is favorable, in the garden.

PAPAYA SKIN

The papaya, an exotic fruit of tropical or semitropical regions, is another unusual source to seek out. It is the inside of ripe papaya skin that should be gently rubbed into the face, elbows, knees or wherever desired. Allow this to remain for at least an hour, then wash off with lukewarm water. This is considered a good skin bracer or astringent.

AVOCADO SKIN OR AVOCADO OIL

The skin of a ripe avocado can be applied in the same manner as the papaya skin. This, as well as the avocado oil, leaves the skin feeling soft and dewey.

VITAMIN E OIL

Liquid Vitamin E is an oil appreciated by many as a miraculous curative balm. Pimples, cuts, skin mutilations and scars are known to be virtually healed with the anointing of Vitamin E.

FACIAL AND BODY PACKS

We know that animals instinctively roll in mud, obviously enjoying this activity. There is therapeutic value in applying moist packs to the body.

In chapter two, "Cosmetic Skin Care," I referred to the facial and body packs formulated by cosmetology specialists. Many of these facial masks are excessively drying to the skin.

There are packs that are beneficial. Some do more than simply soothe and cool the body.

I have formulated a facial pack that is extraordinary in its benefits. It can achieve the following:

1. Unclog pores by softening and dislodging matter that have cluttered the skin.
2. Encourage the free flow of oxygen to promote active breathing of the skin.
3. Healing irritations of the skin.
4. Soothing of nerve endings in the skin.
5. Some tightening of sagging facial muscles.
6. Relaxing some of the tensions or laugh lines in the face.
7. Restore the proper pH balance to the skin.

The ingredients for the mask listed below can be used entirely as one thick application on the face and neck. Or it can be divided for two applications. Because there is no drying to the skin, it can be done frequently.

FACIAL BEAUTY MASK

½ cup oatmeal (uncooked)
1 tablespoon honey (uncooked)
2 tablespoons aloe vera gel
1 teaspoon apple cider vinegar
⅓ to ½ cup of distilled water

Mix together: water, honey, aloe vera gel, and vinegar. Add oatmeal and mix thoroughly. The ingredients should be allowed to set and blend together for at least one hour. For best results, look for a pasty, not watery, consistency. If too dry —stir in a little more distilled water. Place the contents between double thickness of gauze and use as a fascial mask. Allow this to stay on the face from ½ to 1 hour.

You can enjoy the use of these suggested natural ingredients without fear of dangerous side-effects.

Evaluate Your Habits for Skin Beauty

Many habits strongly influence facial appearances. Take stock of some of the focal points on your face.

Are there deep furrows in your forehead, between your brows and above the upper lip?

Lines become etched onto the face with constant frowning and tight-lipped expressions. Without realizing, facial expressions can firmly remain throughout the day and night. Thus a taut, strained look often becomes accepted as a natural part of aging.

You can avoid sculpturing your face with harsh lines by incorporating habits of relaxation.

A few moments of deep breathing, exercised periodically through the day, can help release tight, wound-up feelings of tension. Wipe those lines off your face with deep breathing, especially before dropping off to sleep.

A Good pH Balance Is Necessary

Choose shampoos and soaps that are tested for the proper pH acid balance for skin and hair. A helpful tip in this matter is to add a little apple cider vinegar to your last rinse water when washing the hair. And—add ¼ cup of apple cider vinegar to your bath water.

Do Not Abuse Your Skin

Never apply ice directly to the skin. Blood vessels beneath the skin can be injured this way.

Never squeeze pimples, boils, etc. Infections can result from such forceful procedures, as well as marring the skin with scars. The expulsion of unhealthy or foreign matter from the skin can be encouraged by the use of wet compresses (very warm). Repeat several times a day to achieve quicker results.

I have assembled in this chapter a few of nature's offerings for outside skin care . . . and . . . some guidance in good skin hygiene.

At this point in the book, your common sense can help you understand that outer skin care achievements are very limited. Calling on the natural, wholesome way from within and without, certainly can produce the finest results of a healthy, glowing skin.

Part Six

"HELP FOR DOGS" AND CATS' SKIN AFFLICTIONS

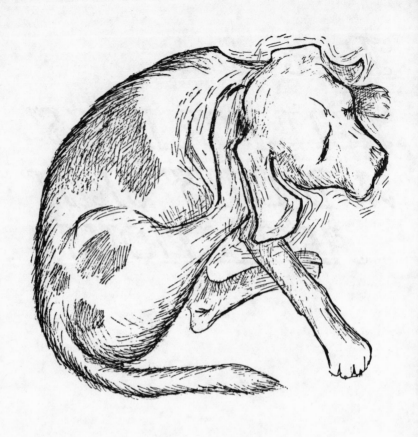

You can help your pet

22.

Pets also have skin problems

What is a chapter on dogs and cats doing in a book about skin? The answer is simple: Many of us have pets and we love them. For this reason, I offer this chapter, as a fringe benefit to all lovers of pets.

History has proven the bodily needs of dogs and cats are quite similar to those of humans. Therefore, I know I can help relieve these animals of much of the nagging skin diseases they endure.

Veterinarians today report they are treating more skin disease than any other ailment. This is mainly owing to the persistence of such disorders —how stubbornly they hang on and on. Many skin disorders of pets seem immune to any medication or treatment. The afflicted pets are subject to constant irritation and discomfort, and owners, too, are distressed because most treatment seems to fail. The situation is painful for the pet and frustrating for the pet owner.

If anything, the problem is on the rise—and becoming unbearable. This is all the more tragic when we consider there are now well over 100 million pet dogs and cats in this country.

Owning a pet brings with it a distinct responsibility. We must make provisions for its well-being; i.e., its feeding, shelter, cleanliness, exercise, and, most of all, its health. Having a pet is no one-sided matter wherein we derive all the pleasure and contribute nothing. Quite the contrary, a pet becomes a member of the family.

Many of the same diseases affect dogs and cats as affect us, and many of their body chemistries are equivalent to ours.

Hair Is an Extension of the Skin

The hair (or fur) of an animal is an extension of the skin. Hair and skin should not be regarded separately. If the fur of an animal is in poor condition, so is the skin, and vice versa. Any infection or parasite which damages the skin will eventually be reflected in the condition of that animal's coat. The condition of the outer coat of a dog or cat is a fairly reliable gauge of that animal's general health.

As with humans, the condition of these external parts of a dog's or cat's body is largely dependent on the nutrition we give it. The balance of health can be tipped, for good or bad, by the quality of the nutrients the animal receives. Even though two-and-one-half billion dollars are spent annually on prepared pet food, I question the nutritive quality of that food, as well as the method in which it is given.

As we go on, it will become apparent that we can do wonders for the health of our pets.

The Dog and the Cat—General Similarities and Dissimilarities

Dogs and cats are similar anatomically and metabolically. Each also has generally the same respiratory, cardiovascular, circulatory, digestive, glandular, and reproductive systems as the other.

The feline eye is somewhat more adaptive than the dog's; the canine's sense of smell is more acute and selective than the cat's. The cat has quicker motor responses, the dog is thought to be more intelligent. As one animal behaviorist has put it, "The chief difference between a dog and cat is that a dog can be taught the meaning of the word 'no.'" Cat lovers, of course, disagree.

Both animals are easily domesticated and seem to thrive in controlled conditions. Each also has considerable capacity to exist in the wild, or semiwild. No amount of domestication completely rids them of instinctual survival responses.

The dog seems less selective in the food it will eat when hungry than is the cat (when equally hungry). Against hostile elements, the dog seems better able to find shelter.

As house pets, the two seem not equatable, since companionship is in the eye of the beholder. If any single generality can be found, it might be that gregarious people like dogs, while more sedate folks prefer the warm, supple grace of a cat.

Whatever their single attributes or failings, the fact remains that dogs and cats bring a certain fullness and satisfaction to the lives of their owners, and, for this, they deserve the best care we can provide.

In the sections which follow, we shall consider each of these highly valued house pets separately.

The Dog

From the Latin Fides (to trust) came the old appellation, Fido. The faithfulness of the dog is legend.

The dog is thought to be the oldest domestic pet. Some years ago, anthropologists unearthed a human skeleton in Africa which was later carbon-dated to at least 80,000 years of age. The skeleton of a dog was with that of the human. While this may not stand as conclusive proof, it suggests the dog has been man's best friend for quite a while.

The Working Dog—The Contributing Dog

The dog has served man in many capacities other than as a pet. He has assisted the shepherd since the dawn of history. He has assisted hunters and pursuers of fugitives just as long. No one can guess how long he has been pulling sleds in the Arctic.

The Dog in Medicine

It was the dog, in fact, upon which vitamins were first tried. In this sense, it can be said the dog has given us the basis for much of our modern theory of nutrition.

Then, too, as everyone knows but cares not to think about, dogs have been used experimentally so that man might learn more about disease. From these practices, however loathesome they may seem to pet lovers, has emerged a great fund of knowledge by which man has learned to live longer and better.

Insulin

The dog, for instance, led us to the discovery of insulin. This was a major medical achievement, for the hard work which led to the eventual control of diabetes did not come easy. After much testing and speculation, a team of Canadian doctors isolated the magic protein, insulin. One of these, a Dr. Charles Best, was the principal recipient of the Nobel Prize in Medicine for this discovery in 1923. But only by means of dogs was the discovery possible.

Anemia

Even before the all-out effort to identify insulin was waged, doctors in California were concerned about the effects of anemia. Somehow, they had to learn more about the body's blood-forming process. Beginning in 1912, countless diets were tested to discover which would best aid in the formation of new, healthy blood. It took thirty years to isolate liver as the singlemost effective natural food in the fight against anemia. Again a Nobel Prize was awarded, and again it was the dog who sacrificed most. But for him, we might not even have this information today.

Rickets

No animal has played a more important role in the prevention of rickets in children than has the dog. Research, reported in medical literature, has been conducted all over the world.

Larger breeds of dogs, such as Great Danes and St. Bernards, are more subject to rickets, primarily because of their rapid growth and large bones.

The work of researchers determined some of the specific causes; deficiencies of calcium and phosphorus in food created bone problems. A diet lacking in calcium and Vitamin D prevented the dog from developing a good skeleton.

This work with dogs finally helped solve the problem of rickets in children.

General Nutrition

All in all, the dog has played an important role in most of the basic discoveries which now underlie the sciences of nutrition and medicine. The processes by which food is converted into bone and muscle are so nearly alike in dog and man that the dog has long been called upon to play a leading role in mankind's expanding medical knowledge. The dog, unlike many other higher animal forms, is able to digest and utilize the same basic foods as man.

The central knowledge we should gain from this is that whatever dietary information we can gain from observing the dog, we should put to use.

The Dog in His Natural Element

Observe the farm dog. Here is nature at her exquisite best.

This dog, by and large, is not fed prepared foods, except perhaps during hard winters. He is often left to fend for himself, not because the owner doesn't care what happens to him, but because the owner knows his dog is resourceful. The farm dog, after killing a rabbit, will eat the whole carcass, even the fur. Especially, he will eat the bones, which contain blood-building marrow.

Unlike the apartment-dwelling city dog, the farm dog has not lost his option to eat raw foods. The farm dog does not have to rely upon meat scraps for protein; his come from the muscles of the rabbit. He does not rely upon bone meal for his calcium and phosphorus; he gets that from the marrow of the rabbit's bones. He is not dependent upon milk products or soybeans for bulk.

The farm dog gets his roughage from the stomach of the rabbit, not from dried corn or wheat products. His vitamins come from the liver of the rabbit.

From these facts we know that farm dogs are eating a completely natural diet—unless and until his owner begins to replace his food. And from simple observation we know that farm dogs are healthier—infinitely healthier—than city-dwelling dogs. They are healthier than the most pampered kennel or show dogs. The farm dog eats as nature intended.

Parallels to Humans

We know that the physiology of dog and man is greatly similar. It has been established many times that whatever is good for a dog also serves man, and vice-versa (I am not suggesting raw, whole rabbits, however). It would seem, then, that humans and canines would suffer roughly the same diseases.

This is only partly true.

Examine the following comparative tables:

COMMON DISEASES OF HUMANS	COMMON DISEASES OF DOGS
HEART DISEASE	HEART DISEASE
INTERNAL CANCERS	INTERNAL CANCERS
EYESIGHT PROBLEMS	EYESIGHT PROBLEMS
ECZEMA	ECZEMA
OSTEOARTHRITIS	OSTEOARTHRITIS
RHEUMATOID ARTHRITIS	
GOUTY ARTHRITIS	NOT COMMON TO
PSORIASIS	THE DOG
GALLSTONES	
SKIN CANCER	

We can see from these tables that humans and dogs suffer some of the same diseases. This is because they share the same habit of drinking oil-free liquids with meals. Habitual use of the water-filled dish alongside the animal's food encourages him to drink at mealtime. In so doing, the dog shares man's habit of consuming an incompatible liquid with food. The diseases shown in the table which apply only to man are owing to his modern "sophistication." He is increasingly tempted with an ever-larger list of adulterated drinks, usually doctored to a chill with ice cubes. Small wonder he is increasingly vulnerable to diseases he would not otherwise acquire.

Unlike the dog, man has "progressed" so far and so fast, he has lost sight of the elemental values of nature.

Factors Other than Liquids

Besides liquids, there are other factors to consider for promoting good health in your pet.

Dr. Clive McCay of Cornell University, in his excellent book, *Nutrition and the Dog*, addresses himself to the relationship between nutrition and disease in dogs.

In this work, he makes a case that good nutrition, far more than drugs, can help the dog ward off disease.

He tells us skin disease bacteria are ever present in the dog and if the animal has a healthy body, there is therefore a strong natural immunity to skin disease. As we said before, the skin is a true barometer which signifies overall health.

McCay found that dietary guidelines were the most important of all considerations in canine health. Vitamins, minerals, and Cod Liver Oil were found to be of ultimate benefit for the dog.

An all-meat or all-fish diet is not ideal, he learned. The deficit of calcium in these heavy protein meals causes crippling bone problems.

McCay found that prevention is the best path for good health, for all living creatures.

Now You Can Be "Dog's Best Friend"

If your dog is healthy, you will want to keep him that way; and if your dog has problems with his skin, you will want to help him. As we have learned from Dr. McCay, this can best be accomplished by improving his eating habits.

Drugs, per se, are not a very satisfactory answer. Many pet owners feel bound to the continuance of the use of drugs when their pets are suffering from mange and other itchy skin infections. If the drug is withheld, they feel, the distressed animal will scratch itself to death.

Sadly, these skin diseases hang on, usually persisting in spite of the drugs.

It is not easy to overcome this problem. We soon develop a feeling of "getting nowhere." We must have courage and perseverance to see our pet through his problem.

With the aid and watchful eye of your veterinarian, you may be able gradually to decrease the use of the medication. And at the same time you should make whatever constructive nutritional changes are necessary.

RULES TO FOLLOW

Liquids

I urge you to control your dog's drinking habits. Have water available most of the time, but, 15 minutes before mealtime, remove it. Do not put water down again until three hours after he has eaten.

Milk is permissible for the dog with or immediately after the meal. I recommend whole milk, since skimmed milk will cause allergies. However, and this is important, milk is to be regarded as a solid food. That is, the dog must not be given water 15 minutes prior to—or within three hours after—the intake of milk.

Cats

I have found, generally, that cats have fewer skin problems than dogs. Cats are by nature dainty eaters and this trait—which carries over into other of the cat's habits, such as its fastidious attention to grooming—best showcases the basic personality difference between dogs and cats.

The cat, as a rule, requires little supervision in feeding. Whereas the dog has a tendency to eat too much, the cat will usually consume only what it needs.

A misconception surrounds milk. Owners have come to believe that milk causes diarrhea (this applies equally to the dog) and therefore have taken to withholding milk from the cat's diet. But it is not whole milk which causes the problem. It is the dry milk solids contained in packaged pet foods which do the actual damage and upset the animal's dietary tract. Elimination of dry milk solids eliminates the diarrhea. But, remember, problems of this nature are not cleared up overnight. Be patient.

Cats are especially fond of fish, but this should not unduly influence selection of their diets. The first dietary rule is to seek balance. An all-fish, or all-meat, diet provides an excess of protein, which in turn can cause kidney problems.

Feeding Dos and Don'ts for Dogs and Cats

1. Base the quantity of food given on the size of the animal. Do not overfeed so that food remains in the bowl. The animal will, in such a case, develop the habit of returning to the bowl and "snacking." The habit of snacking is no more acceptable for pets than for humans. Irregular eating habits are primarily responsible for obesity and resulting poor health.

2. Raw foods are infinitely preferable to prepared foods. This especially applies to eggs, fish, organ meats, etc.

3. Whole milk should always be used. Skimmed milk can create allergies. Dry milk solids are a "fractured food" and create many problems. Only buy prepared pet foods that do not contain dry milk solids, since these create allergies to whole milk.

4. An accelerated good-health regimen is achieved by giving pets a health-food drink. This is made as follows (for a medium-sized dog), and will supply two or three drinks. This can be given as the beginning of a breakfast meal—two or three times a week.

Blend together:

1 tsp. raw wheat germ

6 oz. whole milk

2 raw eggs

½ tsp. whole wheat-germ oil

1 tsp. cold-pressed oil

5. Control water intake of your pet. Do not give water except as instructed in this chapter.

6. Read all prepared-food labels carefully. Avoid all such foods where preservatives and/or milk solids are shown.

7. It is best to adhere to a regular feeding schedule.

8. If you feed your dog table scraps, be sure that you are eating properly.

9. Avoid other than completely natural foods and liquids for your pet. Many people think it is voguish to feed dogs beer, soft drinks, candy, cookies, etc. The animal's body is not equipped to handle such items; they can undermine his health.

Cod Liver Oil

Dosage depends on the size of the pet. A very small animal should receive ¼ teaspoonful. This graduates up to 1 tablespoonful for a very large animal, especially a large dog. This should be given daily until the coat is shiny and evenly textured. Thereafter, give it twice a week for two months, and then once a week.

Generally, it is best if the Cod Liver Oil is stirred into the animal's food. This is most practical because you are dealing with an animal.

The pet should be given the same quality Cod Liver Oil as the owner would take. There is no such thing as a "specially prepared" Cod Liver Oil for pets.

Do not use Cod Liver Oil capsules even though their use seems expedient. Also, the capsulated form of Cod Liver Oil has a tendency to concentrate Vitamins A and D in the animal's liver in too short a time.

Questions and Answers

In the foregoing pages, I have dealt with the general aspects of pet skin care, and have attempted to show that many of the same physical laws that apply to humans also apply to these pets. I have outlined and described the importance of pet diet and care, the need for constant vigilance to be certain they are doing well, and some general information about animal physiology. I hope I have adequately stressed the importance of raw foods, whole milk, Cod Liver Oil, and the timing in which drinking water is given.

But, as stated, the foregoing has been general. Many pet owners have more specific questions in mind. Following is a Question and Answer section, culled from numerous inquiries which have come to me over the years:

Q. Am I wrong in feeding my pet prepared commercial foods?
A. Such foods are unnatural. Commercial pet foods usually contain generous amounts of milk solids, which in turn can cause diarrhea. Read the labels carefully; use those brands with lowest milk-solids content, or with none, if possible. In any event, use prepared foods sparingly. For that matter, it is not difficult to make a mixture of meat and vegetables yourself. You will be doing your pet a favor if you do.

Q. Do you recommend feeding pets scraps from the table?
A. That depends on how you eat. Remember, cats are highly selective, dogs are less so. For instance, dogs dislike sweets (their bodies don't tolerate them well), but if sweets are camouflaged in other foods, the dog will eat them. The real problem here lies in balance and assimilation. If your own diet is balanced, scraps from the table will be fine. In any event, keep a close lookout for changes in the animal's fur. A loss of lustre will indicate the diet is not proper.

Q. Are the cholesterol levels in dogs' and cats' bodies important?
A. Of course. To avoid an unhealthy cholesterol level in your pet, be certain to adhere unfailingly to the instructions given previously in this chapter under the heading "Liquids."

Q. Occasionally my cat—who has the freedom of the back yard —will catch a bird and eat it, feathers and all. Should I keep her indoors to prevent this?
A. Absolutely not. This is instinctual.

Q. Our Collie, who is almost ten years old, is becoming fat. Are reducing diets good for dogs? If so, where can I find one?
A. As with humans, restricted diets for pets can be treacherous, even dangerous. It is vital to achieve and maintain balance. A dog given a normal-portion-for-size diet of natural raw foods and/or health drinks, as well as Cod Liver Oil, will not become overweight unless there is some other specific reason. Very often it is found that inclusion of whole milk

into a dog's diet will alone serve to standardize his weight.

Q. Do spayed and neutered animals have different dietary needs?

A. Definitely. Any operation that alters the natural hormonal balance in any animal body requires that the resulting deficits be compensated for. Such animals need Vitamin E and wheat-germ oil (this latter replaces lost estrogen and prevents excessive shedding).

Q. Are there any specific signs that will tell me my pet needs Cod Liver Oil?

A. Yes. Look for dull, uneven, mottled or discolored fur; scaly tail; dry nose; reddened eyes or any overt signs of arthritis.

Q. How can I keep my dog from shedding?

A. You can't—not altogether. Shedding (the rough equivalent of molting in birds) is common to all animals in some degree. But excessive shedding is abnormal and can be prevented. Both dogs and cats should be given wheat germ oil and wheat germ in their diets when excessive shedding is noted. Also, feed both the germinating seed meals (sesame, sunflower, pumpkin).

Q. How can I recognize a calcium deficiency in my pet?

A. Both cats and dogs exhibit the same symptoms. They are: lack of body in the fur (becomes fine, brittle, silk-thin); twitching of muscles; softening of teeth; swaying of back; splitting nails.

Q. How do I compensate for a calcium deficiency?

A. First of all, the prerequisite steps stated earlier must be taken; that is, inclusion of whole milk and Cod Liver Oil in the diet. Next, fish intake should be increased (this is the best source of phosphorous) for both dogs and cats. Neither animal should be offered any sweets (these days we see faddish pet owners teaching their dogs to drink cola drinks, beer, etc. The dogs invariably develop rheumatoid arthritis.)

Q. I have heard that soy products will cause diarrhea in my dog. Is this so?

A. Yes, because soy products are usually mixed with dry milk solids. If the dog's food comes out of a can, remember also that chemical preservatives must also be dealt with.

Q. Will raw meat harm my dog in any way?

A. None whatever, provided the meat does not contain artificial chemical fatteners such as diethylstilbestrol. Liver is best.

Q. Should fresh bones be part of my dog's diet?

A. Yes, either that or bone meal. But never give a dog chicken bones.

Q. What vitamins are required by cats and dogs?

A. A, B (complex), C, D, E, F, and K. Most of these, of course, are in the natural diet. Vitamin E should be provided all neutered and spayed animals.

Q. Can I substitute irradiated yeast instead of Cod Liver Oil in my pet's food?

A. Try not to. Irradiated yeast is, after all, a synthetic product, and thus unnatural. Use only in emergencies.

Q. If my cat eats a fairly regular fish-based diet, does this mean that I needn't concern myself with additional Cod Liver Oil?

A. No. There is no substitute for Cod Liver Oil.

Part Seven
NEW HORIZONS ON SKIN

23.

New ways
to understand
Your skin

One of the wonders of our age is that we are encouraged to be inquisitive. Not too many years ago, men of medicine were considered to be charlatans, and were watched with a wary eye. Indeed, they often were. Today, physicians are well schooled, and are routinely available.

And yet, for all the medical knowledge which befalls us, there is still some very useful information that seems not to filter down. Let me give you an example: a few days ago I was riding in a car with friends, one of whom was an M.D., and the question was brought up, "What is Sanpaku?" Bob, the doctor, did not know. Now, admittedly, Bob has been away from his practice for a few years (he is writing), but the fact remains that many books have been written on the subject of Sanpaku, and its existence is hardly a secret (Sanpaku is discussed later in this chapter).

Before the term "New Horizon" can have any real significance for us, we must first come to realize that we are very much on our own—health-wise—even in this age of enlightenment. Certainly, we can go to the doctor every time we get a twitch in our little toe, but that's excessive. Trips to the physician should be saved for when they are really needed. Our day-to-day survival is a matter of personal observation and common sense. And so, in a grander sense, is our long-term survival. The "New Horizon" I refer to here is that awareness and vision which will convince you that in the final analysis you are on your own; your body is your castle and you can make it as ugly or as beautiful as you wish it to be. Your health future can be much brighter than you have ever been led to believe.

Your personal skin care will depend largely on your ability to recognize problems early. Much of the information on achieving high-quality, healthy skin is known, and appears in this book, in both general and specific form. The very sad issue is that not even dermatologists today understand the steps required (and available) to make early diagnoses of upcoming skin problems. Obviously, early diagnosis is vitally important. Moreover, the idea of a breakthrough in any medical or related science must deal first with locating and identifying the problem areas. In this respect, any hoped-for "New Horizon" in skin care will be as much diagnostic as anything else.

First, there are a number of signs our body gives us and some of these mean that danger is near, that something serious is already underway. Following is a list of these surface signs that spell D-A-N-G-E-R. The listing which follows deals with six separate areas of the body: the tongue, the eyes, the face, the ear, the beard, and the hair. All of these are "skin" areas, and each tells a specific story. Remember, above all else, that the appearance and condition of the skin is a cash-register total of all your previous mistakes.

The Tongue

The tongue (remember, the tongue is part of the skin) is a dependable barometer of general health. The classic sign has heretofore been limited to "coating" without respect to color, serrated edges, etc. All these things tell us a message. These signs, in effect, are the body's dietary printout.

The following list includes most of the classic

BACK OF TONGUE BROWNING INDICATES LIVER OR GALL BLADDER PROBLEM

GREENISH COATING INDICATES CONSTIPATION

SERRATED EDGE INDICATES BODY'S TOLERANCE OF SWEETS HAS BEEN EXCEEDED

CENTER FISSURE INDICATES PROTEIN IMBALANCE

MAPLIKE FISSURES INDICATE MINERAL IMBALANCE

RAW RED TIP INDICATES VITAMIN DEFICIENCY

NERVOUS TONGUE INDICATES NERVOUS DISORDER

The tongue is also a dependable barometer of general health

symptoms considered by many to be valid and useful diagnostic tools.

A. The *Serrated-Edge* tongue tells us a lot. The serration tells us that the body's tolerance for sweets has been exceeded. The amount of serration tells us to what degree this is so. If the serration is accompanied by inflammation on the top-edge of the tongue, a very serious problem is indicated. If the tongue is ulcerated-appearing or "creviced," the body is objecting just about as loudly as it can.

B. The *Center-Fissure* tongue indicates a protein imbalance. Geographical (maplike) fissures suggest a mineral imbalance. Grooves or fissures anywhere on the tongue indicate the body is not assimilating protein or minerals properly.

C. A coating of greenish hue indicates constipation.

D. A raw, red tip indicates a vitamin deficiency.

E. If the back of the tongue is *browning*, a gallbladder or liver problem exists. Sometimes, however, heavy smokers can develop a "brown" tongue which is indicative of no dietary shortcoming.

F. The *Nervous Tongue* tells us perhaps the most dire news of all. Those who cannot hold their tongue out and *completely motionless* are suffering a nervous disorder. If the tongue waves back and forth uncontrollably, an impending nervous breakdown is suspect.

The Physiognomy (*the face*)

A. *Pores.* No one is born with large pores. Pores usually become enlarged at an early age, very often caused by a preponderance of sweets. Once enlarged, pores will not regain their normal size. Large pores are never caused by external abuse—they are the perfect telltale sign of poor diet. Enlargement begins on the cheeks and spreads to the nose and forehead. Enlarged pores should be looked for constantly in the young, and, when occurring, should lead to a change of diet immediately. Blackheads and whiteheads are a secondary sign of enlarged pores, and primarily have very little to do with hygiene. Pimples are an indication that the skin has been flooded with sugary liquids (as opposed to the sweets found in cakes or pies, which sugar is chewed). When sugary liquids are drunk on an empty stomach, pimples are just a matter of time.

The Eyes

A. *Swelling under the eyes* (bags) indicate an electrolyte imbalance. It is usually corrected (if not too far gone) by removing salt from the diet and by eating raw salads. Usually beginning in the twenty-forty age bracket, "bags" are often correctly associated with liquor consumption, especially liquor consumption *with*

food, and more especially yet if the habit
of drinking alcohol with meals is started
early in life. Ice water with meals is another contributor to this condition.

B. *Crow's Feet.* Lateral or "rayed" lines
projecting from the outer corner of the
eye indicate the skin is losing its elasticity.
This is usually traceable to a heavy intake
of tannic acid, and is aggravated by sun-
squinting.

C. *Frown lines and Smile lines.* These are
accelerated early in life by choice of vo-
cation. Actors, for instance, are encouraged to exaggerate facial expressions. Diet
enters the picture only after the choice of
career has set the lines. A poor diet will
serve to set the lines all the deeper.

D. *Chelazians.* Smallish, yellow-whitish
growths (but not of a malignant nature)
in the inner corner of the eyes. Caused by
calcinosis, owing to improper regulation
of calcium in the diet.

E. *Sanpaku* (from the Japanese: San = three
and Paku = white sides; hence, three visible areas of white around the iris). The
normal eye, looking straight ahead and
with muscles relaxed, will display visible
white only at the sides. When white is also
visible *below* the iris, mental deteriora-

tion is evident, mental breakdown is around the corner, and suicidal tendencies become common. Japanese scientists have concluded that Sanpaku is related to diets leaning heavily to refined foods and overcooking. It is no mere play on words to say that white sugar can lead to insanity.

The Ear

The deep-creased earlobe indicates a predisposition to heart disease. It has been theorized this is owing to a loss of elasticity in the lobe, probably caused by improper oil metabolism.

The Beard

The beard is an excellent indicator of the body's mineral metabolism. An evenly-colored beard is an indication that your mineral balance is good. A multi-colored beard (especially, a beard which is white in the center) indicates a mineral deficiency.

The Hair

A. A receding hairline indicates that germination and estrogen factors are inadequate. Normal wear and tear (caused by sleeping position, tight hats, etc.) and/or circulation problems account for specific baldness, but a uniformly receding hairline indicates dietary imbalance. You need germinating foods: raw wheat germ, raw onion, sunflower seeds. Wheat germ oil and raw eggs provide estrogen.

B. Grey or white hair is determined by a preponderance of acid-bearing liquids in the diet. Much is governed by the age at which you begin drinking them. High concentrations of acid-bearing liquids (especially frozen juices) can produce streaks of white.

The Hand

The back of the hand is as interesting to the scientist as is the palm to the fortuneteller. The reason the hand is such a good barometer is that the tissues are soft and register dietary mistakes more quickly. *Angry veins* (wide, narrow, sclerosed, bulbous) indicate veins are not adequately supported by fatty tissue (this was a common symptom which resulted in released concentration camp victims). Long-term fasting, followed by resumption of a normal diet, is also responsible. *Furrowed spacing between ligaments* indicates a negative protein balance (the body is using its own proteins). This is a mark of anyone who drinks improper liquids with meals, or who is protein starved. Often this is corroborated by a fissure in the center of the tongue. *Brown pigmentations* (often called *Liver Spots*) are the result of B-Complex deficiency. Long term use of sweets or ice cream (except homemade) accounts for much of this. *Half-moon loss* in the fingernails indicates a Vitamin C deficiency. The *Washboard Effect* across the thumbnail indicates too much carbonated soft drinks begun too early in life.

In Closing

None of the foregoing information is new. Casual conversations among food-faddists have always centered about general symptomatology as it might relate to dietary questions and answers, and, often, their suspicions have had some basis in fact. But finding the true character and reason for such symptoms remained for the scientists to uncover. And scientists, as we have learned, are not always quick to let us know what they know. To find out about Sanpaku or ridged thumbnails, for example, one would have had to make a probing examination of medical literature.

These guidelines have been included here because they are valuable, not just because they are conversational. These few atypical symptoms can be every bit as valuable as the symptoms which indicate appendicitis, and thereby save your life. Any thinking person should know enough to take advantage of them. Do not regard them as mere symbols or talismans or the work of some hereditary devil. They are much more than that. They are warning sirens. Your body is screaming for corrective action.

And thus I offer the reader a New Horizon. From this point forward, he need no longer be puzzled by the simple physical language of nature. When the sign is present, he can take the steps indicated and build his personal castle of life into a more permanent house, or he can do as he has always done and pay the price.

The difference is that he now has an option.

Part Eight

THE SURE WAY TO HEALTHY SKIN

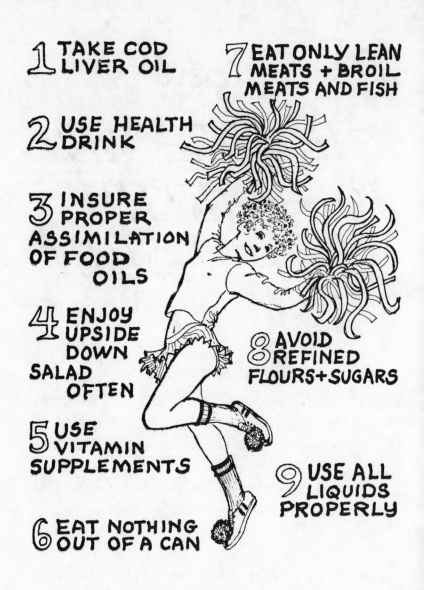

1 TAKE COD LIVER OIL

2 USE HEALTH DRINK

3 INSURE PROPER ASSIMILATION OF FOOD OILS

4 ENJOY UPSIDE DOWN SALAD OFTEN

5 USE VITAMIN SUPPLEMENTS

6 EAT NOTHING OUT OF A CAN

7 EAT ONLY LEAN MEATS + BROIL MEATS AND FISH

8 AVOID REFINED FLOURS + SUGARS

9 USE ALL LIQUIDS PROPERLY

Here's to a happy way of life

24

Nine special rules to live by

The success or failure of any undertaking is tied directly to the enthusiasm, purpose, and diligence of the one involved. This is true of tangible things, such as succeeding at business, and intangible things as well, such as achieving happiness. One's frame of mind has everything to do with the eventual results.

Your purpose in having gone this far in this book should be directly linked to your desire to have good health—especially as is manifest in the condition of the skin. Your investment, in both time and money, is now ready to pay off. Nothing stands in the way, provided you now bring the whole matter to fruition, and provided you do so with a predetermined conviction that you can and will succeed. In a word, you must fire your enthusiasm, and then sustain it. This book, like all others, will be only as useful as you make it. You

301

now have all the information you need to start on the road to good health, and especially good skin health.

The condition of our skin tells the story of our lives. In many cases, we can almost chronicle the way a person has lived his life by looking at his skin, since the condition of the skin reflects the extent to which he has been a victim of habit. If a bad habit has been long-ingrained, it will be very difficult to break; if skin-abuse has been long established, it will be quite difficult to alter. Recently dried-out skin is much easier to deal with than is long-established dryness. If that dryness has been lifelong, it will be very difficult to change. Everything will depend on the amount of scar tissue which has been formed—how much damage has been done to the sebaceous ducts, and how much they have atrophied.

But there is virtually no condition of the skin which cannot be improved in some degree by adherence to the simple but explicit rules which follow:

The Nine Primary Rules of Skin Care

Rule One:
Take Cod Liver Oil in the precise manner outlined in this book. Cod Liver Oil is the primary moisturizer and elasticizer.

Rule One is critical. You determine, with employment of this rule, just how effective will be your fight. The greater the intensity of consistent Cod Liver Oil intake (up to a point), the faster will be the rate of improvement you will see. Daily Cod Liver Oil use for the first six months may be indicated if the hair is very dry or brittle, since the hair will make a greater demand upon the available oil than will the skin. If the hair is in good condition, the oil will be immediately available to the skin, and improvement will be seen faster.

In any event, whether taken daily or weekly, Cod Liver Oil will hasten the effects you seek. Most skin shortcomings should improve in six months if you faithfully combine a Cod Liver Oil regimen with good eating habits. Remember, no capsules.

Rule Two:

Use the Health Drink. Six months regular usage of this greatly important dietary tool will make all the difference. For the first six months, take the health drink daily, substituting for breakfast or lunch in the regular diet. Take it once a week after that.

The health drink is, when properly and selectively made, using only raw and enzyme-rich nutrients, one of the greatest promoters of glowing skin. Through the health drink is achieved a youthful, rejuvenated appearance. This is because the health drink is rich in B-Complex vitamins, unsaturated fatty acids, Vitamin C, and minerals.

Rule Three:

Rule three concerns proper assimilation of liquids, as earlier described in this book. You can easily shortchange yourself if you drink the wrong liquids, or even the correct liquids at the wrong time. Never use ice.

Proper assimilation ensures lubricant control of the body. The vitaminless oils can then do their job properly (which is to supply energy) and the oils containing vitamins can do theirs (provide lubrication).

Usually, you can tell if your body is assimilating fuels properly simply by the "warmth" and "comfort" of your extremities. Cold hands and/or feet indicate poor circulation, principally owing to an improper assimilation of oils.

Rule Four:

Make it a point to eat the Upside-Down Salad as often as possible. Twice a day is not too much. The ingredients of this salad provide for purification of the skin. That "alive" color, especially in the cheeks, is achieved in this manner.

There is no reason to believe the Upside-Down Salad need ever become a dietary drudge. It can be made in at least fifty different ways. With substitutions of fish, meat, nuts, eggs, fruit, raisins, etc., the Upside-Down Salad can become a convertible delight. The only absolute conditions are that the salad contain a proper oil (or oils), and herbs. Vegetable salads are greatly preferable to others, but you needn't limit yourself to them. Give your taste buds a chance.

Rule Five:

Use Vitamin Supplements. This is greatly important if we cook our foods. Remember that cooking, even a moderate amount of it, destroys vitamins, minerals, and enzymes. The less you cook, the less you will be dependent upon vitamin supplements.

Habitual cooking of food accelerates the aging process. A "naturally paced" aging process results only from constant intake of useful, natural vitamins, minerals, and enzymes, but certain deficiencies in this area can be offset by sensible use of supplements.

Remember that organic (natural) vitamins are greatly preferable to the synthetic because their intrinsic factors are intact.

But don't assume that taking vitamins will solve all the problems. Wholesome nutrition is of primary importance.

Rule Six:

Eat nothing out of a can. In the course of canning, most of the life has been extracted from the food. The heat from processing has roughly the same effect upon food as does a lit match upon dry tinder. Moreover, the additives and preservatives used to ensure shelf-life are of such a nature as to compound the natural problems of the body. Canned foods, generally, are constipating.

Canned foods can be likened to the candy bar; they provide short-term energy—nothing else. We have been sold on the ideas that (1) canned foods represent a basic economy since they are cheap to produce, and (2) by virtue of cans, we may have certain fruits and vegetables out of season. Well, the economy alluded to is false, and the selection of natural foodstuffs is bountiful enough to please any palate, if we make wise choices. Nobody needs strawberries in December.

Rule Seven:

Eat only **LEAN** meats, and **BROIL** all meats and fish. Natural meat fats are saturated fats and are exceptionally difficult for the body to handle. Avoid them. Frying with oil destroys the value of the food (good oils become worthless, and bad oils become worse).

Fish is superior to all other flesh-foodstuffs. Whole civilizations have survived on fish. Just as vegetables are kings among the edible flora, so too are fish king among the fauna. Besides, with the exception of insects, there are probably more fish than anything else on this planet; eating them seems an ecological plus.

Rule Eight:

Avoid refined flours and sugars. In fact, avoid them like a plague.

Since time began, man has been doing things that seemed useful to him. That has been his rationale for both wars and commerce. It is debatable whether he has been more foolish in his wars or in his commerce, for he has committed enormous blunders in the name of each.

The early commerce of the Hawaiian Islands was limited to the export of pineapples and cane sugar. Early shippers complained they could not carry enough raw cane to make a profitable trip to the States. Hence the evolution of "refining." By boiling the cane and then dehydrating the residue, "sugar" was produced. Bleaching made it white, which color symbolized "purity." Roughly the same story surrounds the milling of wheat and its transformation into bleached, white flour.

In either case, the natural foodstuff has been rendered almost worthless, and must not be used. Such refined foods retard healthy bacterial growth in the human intestine, and thus are a hindrance in the formation of what is called "intestinal flora." A secondary result is that the normal peristaltic action of the intestines is reduced, causing constipation.

Permit yourself only a minimum of sweets. Natural sweets are allowed (dates, figs, raisins, fresh fruits, etc.).

Rule Nine:

<u>Use all liquids properly.</u> Everything depends on the proper intake of liquids. Remember that milk and homemade soups are the only oil-bearing liquids permitted with

meals. Water is allowed not less than 10 minutes before a meal, nor less than three hours afterward.

The foregoing nine rules are designed to give you an easy-to-remember "system" by which you can avail yourself of general good health—and correspondingly high-quality skin in a minimum of time. If you follow these rules faithfully, and err as little as possible, your life should undergo some noticeable changes. Not only will your general health and skin tone improve, but so should your whole life. Being healthier and looking better cannot help but alter your appreciation of yourself and, thus, your relationships with others. You will be more fun to be around, and so the social structure of your existence will also improve. My nine rules are actually nine rules to happiness.

SEND A COPY TO A FRIEND

Here you have an opportunity to do a good deed for a friend in need. Until now, there has never been a book on skin care written more clearly . . . showing the sure-fire way to better skin health. It tells about the method that really works—to approach the skin problem from the inside—not from the outside cosmetic way.

For additional copies we suggest you first try your local bookstores or department stores. If they happen to be out of stock we will be pleased to receive your orders directly, and they will be shipped immediately, postpaid. The price is $8.95 plus .50¢ postage and handling. Include a letter with your address, or the address of the person you want to receive the book. Send to:

THE WITKOWER PRESS, INC.
Box 2296, Bishops Corner
West Hartford, Conn. 06117

—OTHER BOOKS BY DALE ALEXANDER—
ARTHRITIS AND COMMON SENSE
GOOD HEALTH AND COMMON SENSE
COMMON COLD AND COMMON SENSE
HEALTHY HAIR AND COMMON SENSE
All books $8.95 + .50¢ handling charge each.

INDEX

Acne, 4, 52, 87–91
  diet and, 88–91, 99, 102, 250, 251
  emotions and, 105
Acne Rosacea, 108
Adler, Alfred, 103
Aging, Prevention, 244–245
Albinos, 45–46
Allergies, 169–170, 251
  See also Diets, Balanced
American Journal of Diseases of Children, 137
American Practitioner's Transaction, 149
Andelman, Dr. S. L., 92–93
Archives of Internal Medicine, 136
Arthritis, 38, 129–134, 136–137
Arthritis and Common Sense, 5–6, 131–132
Atkins, Dr. Robert, 117–118
Awareness, Developing, 288–289

Bacon, Francis, 18
Bacteriology, 20
Bad breath, 145
Baldness, 53
Baths, 9
Beard as diagnostic aid, 294
Best, Dr. Charles, 270
Biochemical individuality, 101–102
Blackheads, 73, 250–251
Brown University, 25
Buckley, Dr. L. Duncan, 130

Canadian Medical Association, 239
Cancer, 52–53
  earwax and, 147–148
Cancer (skin), 4, 99–102, 250
  Australian incidence, 100
  dietary causes, 100, 250
Cats. *See* Pets, Skin problems
Cheraskin, Dr. E., 209–210
Cholesterol, 109, 113–127, 231–232
  assimilation, 121–128
  description, 113–114
  diet, 116–119, 120–123
  effect of cod liver oil on, 137–138
  heart disease and, 116–120
  See also Margarine
Cleopatra, 4, 9
Cod liver oil, 60–67, 81, 102, 128–142, 149, 153, 217, 250, 275, 280, 302–304
  appearance in medical texts, 136
  effect on cholesterol, 137–138
  effect on earwax, 149, 153
  for arthritis, 129–134
  for eczema, 94
  for psoriasis, 95–99
  for skin cancer, 101
  history of use, 132–140
  milkshakes, 63–65, 250
  Norwegian variety, 135
  pets, 275, 280
  See also Diets, Balanced
Constipation. *See* Regularity
Cornell University, 212